Options for Surgical Exposure and Soft Tissue Coverage in Upper Extremity Trauma

Editor

AMITAVA GUPTA

HAND CLINICS

www.hand.theclinics.com

Consulting Editor
KEVIN C. CHUNG

November 2014 • Volume 30 • Number 4

ELSEVIER

1600 John F. Kennedy Boulevard • Suite 1800 • Philadelphia, Pennsylvania, 19103-2899

http://www.theclinics.com

HAND CLINICS Volume 30, Number 4
November 2014 ISSN 0749-0712, ISBN-13: 978-0-323-32375-8

Editor: Jennifer Flynn-Briggs
Developmental editor: Stephanie Carter

Hand Clinics (ISSN 0749-0712) is published quarterly by Elsevier Inc., 360 Park Avenue South, New York, NY 10010-1710. Months of publication are February, May, August, and November. Business and Editorial Offices: 1600 John F. Kennedy Blvd., Ste. 1800, Philadelphia, PA 19103-2899. Customer Service Office: 3251 Riverport Lane, Maryland Heights, MO 63043. Periodicals postage paid at New York, NY and at additional mailing offices. Subscription price is $390.00 per year (domestic individuals), $606.00 per year (domestic institutions), $194.00 per year (domestic students/residents), $445.00 per year (Canadian individuals), $691.00 per year (Canadian institutions), $530.00 per year (international individuals), $691.00 per year (international institutions), and $256.00 per year (international and Canadian students/residents). Foreign air speed delivery is included in all *Clinics* subscription prices. All prices are subject to change without notice. **POSTMASTER:** Send address changes to *Hand Clinics*, Elsevier Health Sciences Division, Subscription Customer Service, 3251 Riverport Lane, Maryland Heights, MO 63043. Customer Service (orders, claims, online, change of address): Elsevier Health Sciences Division, Subscription Customer Service, 3251 Riverport Lane, Maryland Heights, MO 63043. Tel: 1-800-654-2452 (U.S. and Canada); 314-447-8871 (outside U.S. and Canada). Fax: 314-447-8029. E-mail: journalscustomerservice-usa@elsevier.com (for print support); journalsonlinesupport-usa@elsevier.com (for online support).

Reprints. For copies of 100 or more of articles in this publication, please contact the Commercial Reprints Department, Elsevier Inc., 360 Park Avenue South, New York, New York 10010-1710. Tel.: 212-633-3874; Fax: 212-633-3820; E-mail: reprints@elsevier.com.

Hand Clinics is covered in *MEDLINE/PubMed (Index Medicus), Current Contents/Clinical Medicine, EMBASE/Excerpta Medica,* and *ISI/BIOMED.*

Contributors

CONSULTING EDITOR

KEVIN C. CHUNG, MD, MS
Chief of Hand Surgery, University of Michigan
Health System; Charles B. G. de Nancrede
Professor of Surgery, Section of Plastic
Surgery, Department of Surgery; Professor of
Orthopaedic Surgery; Assistant Dean for
Faculty Affairs; Associate Director of Global
REACH, Ann Arbor, Michigan

EDITOR

AMITAVA GUPTA, MD, FRCS
Director, Louisville Arm and Hand, Louisville,
Kentucky

AUTHORS

TERRY S. AXELROD, MD, MSc, FRCSC
Professor of Surgery, Division of Orthopaedic
Surgery, University of Toronto, Ontario,
Canada

KYLE D. BICKEL, MD
The Hand Center of San Francisco, San
Francisco, California

PAUL BINHAMMER, MSc, MD, FRCS(C)
Assistant Professor, Division of Plastic
Surgery, University of Toronto, Toronto,
Ontario, Canada

JOHN T. CAPO, MD
Professor, Department of Orthopaedics, NYU
Langone Medical Center, NYU Hospital for
Joint Diseases, New York, New York

BRIAN T. CARLSEN, MD
Division of Plastic Surgery, Mayo Clinic,
Rochester, Minnesota

HARVEY CHIM, MD
Division of Plastic Surgery, University of Miami
Miller School of Medicine, Miami, Florida

KEVIN C. CHUNG, MD, MS
Chief of Hand Surgery, University of Michigan
Health System; Charles B. G. de Nancrede
Professor of Surgery, Section of Plastic
Surgery, Department of Surgery; Professor of
Orthopaedic Surgery; Assistant Dean for
Faculty Affairs; Associate Director of Global
REACH, Ann Arbor, Michigan

KATHARINE T. CRINER, MD
Hand Fellow, Division of Hand Surgery,
Department of Orthopaedics, NYU Hospital
for Joint Diseases, New York, New York

AMITAVA GUPTA, MD, FRCS
Director, Louisville Arm and Hand, Louisville,
Kentucky

HARRY HOYEN, MD
Associate Professor, Department of
Orthopaedic Surgery, MetroHealth Medical
Center, Case Western Reserve University,
Cleveland, Ohio

MELISSA A. KLAUSMEYER, MD
Assistant Professor, Division of Plastic and
Reconstructive Surgery, Department of
Orthopedic Surgery, University of Colorado
Hospital, Aurora, Colorado

ANITA T. MOHAN, MD
Division of Plastic Surgery, Mayo Clinic,
Rochester, Minnesota

CHAITANYA MUDGAL, MD
Assistant Professor, Hand and Upper
Extremity Service, Department of Orthopedics,
Harvard Medical School, Boston,
Massachusetts

ZHI YANG NG, MRCS
Department of Plastic Reconstructive and
Aesthetic Surgery, Singapore General
Hospital, Singapore

RICK PAPENDREA, MD
Clinical Assistant Professor, Department of
Orthopaedic Surgery, Medical College of
Wisconsin, Milwaukee, Wisconsin; Papendrea

Orthopaedic Associates of Wisconsin,
Waukesha, Wisconsin

MICHEL SAINT-CYR, MD
Division of Plastic Surgery, Mayo Clinic,
Rochester, Minnesota

BEN SHAMIAN, MD
Resident, Department of Medicine,
NYU Woodhull Medical Center, Brooklyn,
New York

ANDREW J. WATT, MD
Attending Surgeon, Department of Plastic
Surgery, The Buncke Clinic, California
Pacific Medical Center, San Francisco,
California; Adjunct Clinical Faculty, Division
of Plastic and Reconstructive Surgery,
Stanford University School of Medicine,
Stanford, California

ZACH YENNA, MD
Resident, Department of Orthopedic
Surgery, University of Louisville, Louisville,
Kentucky

Contents

Extensile and adequate exposures of the shoulder and upper humerus are important in trauma surgery. The standard deltopectoral approach can be extended distally to expose the whole humerus if necessary. Often, wide exposures of the upper humerus are necessary to reduce complex fractures and apply the plate on the lateral aspect of the humerus. A thorough knowledge of the anatomy as well as strategies of nerve mobilization is necessary for achieving adequate exposures in this area. This article details the many exposure methods for the shoulder, upper humerus, and their extensile extensions.

The care of humeral shaft fractures is undergoing a transition to more aggressive treatment methods with more frequent operative fixation. The upper arm has an extensive network of nerves, arteries, and veins that must be protected during any operative exposure. The ultimate goal of fixation of a humerus fracture is rigid stabilization to allow early range of motion, protection of the neurovascular structures, and preservation of the triceps mechanism posteriorly and the anterior elbow flexor muscles.

This article describes the basic bony, ligamentous, and neurologic anatomy of the structures about the elbow. The surgical exposures of the elbow joint are described, providing details of the various posterior, lateral, and medial approaches to the articular segments. Clinical applications describing the potential benefits of each surgical exposure are provided as examples.

Approaches to the forearm use internervous planes to allow adequate bone exposure and prevent muscle denervation. The Henry approach utilizes the plane between muscles supplied by the median and radial nerves. The Thompson approach utilizes the plane between muscles supplied by the radial and posterior interosseous nerves. The distal radius may be approached volarly. The extended flexor carpi radialis approach is useful for intraarticular fractures, subacute fractures, and malunions. The distal radius can be approached dorsally by releasing the third dorsal compartment and continuing the dissection subperiosteally. Choice of approach depends on the injury pattern and the need for exposure.

debitating. The hand has evolved into a complex, intricate structural conglomeration of bones, joints, tendons, ligaments, and neurovascular structures, with an overlying soft tissue envelope that is varied and adapted to particular functions. Wounds to the hand requiring flap coverage warrant careful planning. Increasing knowledge of anatomy has led to the description of many flaps. This article presents a review of the commonly used flaps in reconstruction of the hand and the various considerations involved.

HAND CLINICS

Preface

Options for Surgical Exposure and Soft Tissue Coverage in Upper Extremity Trauma

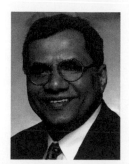

Amitava Gupta, MD, FRCS
Editor

My friend and teacher, Robert Acland, MD, has two famous sayings that are very relevant to the current issue of the *Hand Clinics*. The first is: "Preparation is the only shortcut you will ever need." The second is: "the anatomical structures are under no moral obligation to be where you think they should be. They are where they are."

The first saying emphasizes the importance of planning in surgical procedures. The second outlines the importance of anatomic knowledge, especially the appreciation of anatomic variability.

For a surgeon, knowledge of anatomy is of the utmost importance. Jean Cruveilhier, in his 1834 treatise *Anatomie Descriptive*, said, "There is no surgery, physiology or medicine without anatomy." In this issue, we have concentrated on the anatomic basis of exposures and coverage of the upper extremity with tips and tricks to help the surgeon along with clinical examples where appropriate.

In the first section, we have attempted to provide a comprehensive description of standard and alternative exposures of the shoulder, arm, elbow, forearm, and hand along with the relevant anatomy, pearls, and pitfalls of the described exposures and case examples illustrating the relevant points.

The focus of the second section is on soft tissue coverage of the upper extremity, discussing the standard methods along with alternatives illustrated with relevant clinical examples.

The authors of the individual articles are all experts in their fields and have vast experience in surgery and surgical teaching. I am very grateful to them for sharing their knowledge and experience with us.

I am humbled by the opportunity to be the Guest Editor of this issue of *Hand Clinics*. For this honor, I would like to thank Kevin Chung, MD, who is the Consulting Editor of *Hand Clinics*. My full appreciation to the editorial staff of the *Hand Clinics*, especially Ms Stephanie Carter, for all the help and support that I and the other authors have received.

Amitava Gupta, MD, FRCS
Director, Louisville Arm and Hand
Louisville, KY 40202, USA

E-mail address:
armhand@gmail.com

Hand Clin 30 (2014) ix
http://dx.doi.org/10.1016/j.hcl.2014.08.004

Exposures of the Shoulder and Upper Humerus

Harry Hoyen, MD[a],*, Rick Papendrea, MD[b]

KEYWORDS

- Anterior exposure • Anterolateral exposure • Posterior exposure • Extensile Judet exposure
- Deltopectoral • Axillary nerve • Radial nerve

KEY POINTS

- The standard exposure to the shoulder and upper humerus is through a deltopectoral approach.
- Strategies for mobilization of the deltoid and exposure of the axillary nerve are important for wider exposure of the proximal humerus.
- Extensile approaches enable exposure of the whole humerus.

INTRODUCTION

The surgical approaches to the shoulder and upper humerus are essential for the trauma and reconstructive surgeon. The ability to perform a facile exposure to the upper arm will pay dividends in arthroplasty and fracture stabilization procedures. Owing to the intricate relationship between the vital neurovascular structures, muscle envelope, and necessary osseous exposure; minimally invasive procedures are not utilized or as necessary as with the lower limb.

The basic principles for exposure depend on the primary placement of the fixation. Although this article does not discuss in great detail primary arthroplasty procedures, in complex trauma, hemiarthroplasty, and reverse arthroplasty for proximal humerus fractures may be necessary. Thus, the choice of exposure in fractures that require an intraoperative decision between arthroplasty and fixation is vitally important.

In general terms, fixation is located along the lateral part of the upper humerus, with distal fixation in the posterior region. In the shoulder region, the approach is through a traditional anterior exposure or anterolateral approach. **Fig. 1** shows the different approaches to the shoulder.

Although this article has some overlap with the fixation technique article for the humerus (see the discussion by Capo, Criner, and Shamian, also in this issue), this can be used as a guide to determine which fracture patterns are amendable to each exposure type. The tips for exposure are described with the advantages and disadvantages highlighted. The majority of these approaches are through predictable internervous planes.

ANTERIOR SHOULDER EXPOSURE
Deltopectoral

The traditional anterior shoulder exposure or the workhorse for arthroplasty and fixation has been the deltopectoral exposure. The incision is center of the deltoid–pectoral interval, which is typically over the coracoid. The swelling in the shoulder after trauma can make it difficult to identify the

[a] Department of Orthopaedic Surgery, MetroHealth Medical Center, Case Western Reserve University, 2500 Metrohealth Drive, Cleveland, OH 44109, USA; [b] Department of Orthopaedic Surgery, Medical College of Wisconsin, Papendrea Orthopaedic Associates of Wisconsin, S.C. 1111 Delafield Street, Suite 120, Waukesha, WI 53188, USA
* Corresponding author.
E-mail address: hhoyen@metrohealth.org

Hand Clin 30 (2014) 391–399
http://dx.doi.org/10.1016/j.hcl.2014.08.003
0749-0712/14/$ – see front matter © 2014 Elsevier Inc. All rights reserved.

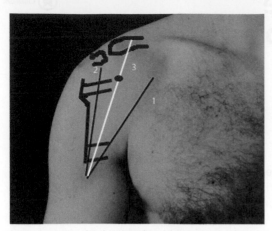

Fig. 1. Anterior skin landmarks with depiction of lateral plate fixation. (1) Actual interval between the deltoid and pectoralis muscles. (2) Interval between the anterior and middle portions of the deltoid. (3) Incision for the deltopectoral approach.

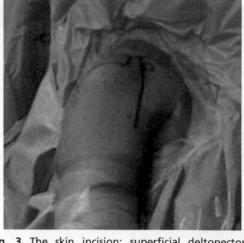

Fig. 3. The skin incision: superficial deltopectoral interval.

medial aspect of the deltoid, thus keeping the exposure toward the more palpable coracoid (**Fig. 2**).

Whether it is the anterior exposure to the glenohumeral joint for arthroplasty or the lateral aspect of the proximal humerus, the deltoid shrouds the exposure (**Figs. 3** and **4**). There are several strategies for mobilizing the deltoid. The distal aspect of the deltoid and the anterior aspect of its tendinous insertion can be mobilized to permit lateral retraction of the deltoid. There are multiple perforating

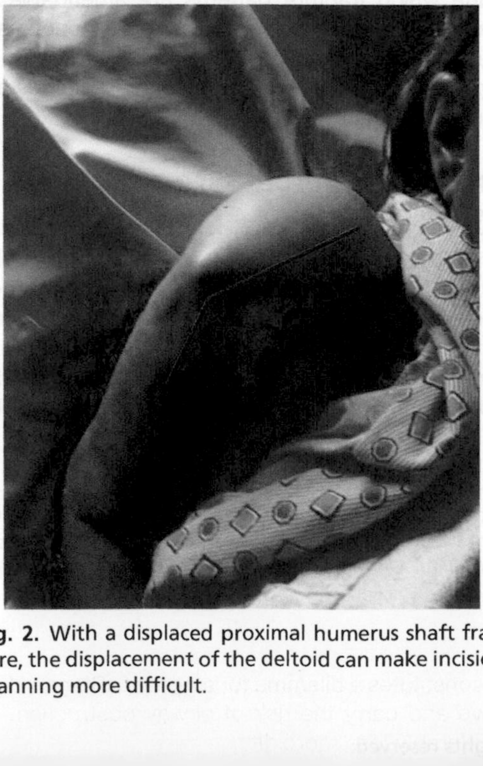

Fig. 2. With a displaced proximal humerus shaft fracture, the displacement of the deltoid can make incision planning more difficult.

vessels at the anterior deltoid insertion that require bovie electrocautery. The deltoid insertion is quite encompassing around the posterior aspect of the humerus and the anterior fibers and periosteum can be elevated without concern of proximal migration of the muscle. This enables the entire anterior muscle tendon unit to be mobilized laterally.

The clavipectoral fascia is cleared to identify the rotator cuff interval and subacromial space. There is a definitive, palpable separation between the supraspinatus and subscapularis. If the surgeon cannot identify the rotator interval, the biceps tendon in the bicipital groove can be followed proximal to the distal edge of the anterior supraspinatus fibers. These fibers are very stout, but slightly posterior and medial dissection will lead to the interval (**Fig. 5A**).

As the biceps exits the groove distally, the inferior border of the subscapularis can be palpated. This will lead to proximal humerus calcar and the axillary nerve as it courses beneath the inferior capsule. Although the calcar cannot be directly visualized, the reduction cannot be palpated through this exposure. The axillary nerve can be palpated underneath the conjoined tendon. It is in very close proximity and courses just beneath the glenohumeral joint capsule.

The axillary nerve can also be found laterally as it is arborizing within the deltoid. Another important fracture landmark is that the nerve is often found at the distal spike of the greater tuberosity fragment. It is helpful to mobilize the nerve from this spike and the humerus. This is important for later fracture reduction, because this distal spike can often be anatomically reduced. This move will

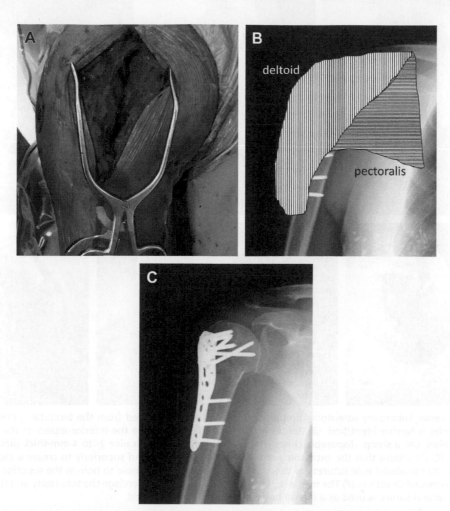

Fig. 4. (*A, B*) Deltoid and pectoralis muscles envelop the proximal humerus. (*C*) Even though the exposure, the plate is applied to the lateral humerus with fixation.

provide reestablishment of the greater tuberosity height. The humeral head needs to be elevated and reduced to this position, rather than reducing the tuberosities to the humeral head.

A difficult part of the reduction of the surgical neck portion of the proximal humerus fracture is that external rotation is necessary for fracture reduction but the plate application is more difficult owing to the deltoid. The screw fixation is applied first distally as the tendon can be retracted. Anterior wire fixation with the plate in situ or along the anterior cortex can permit enough fixation such that the arm can be internally rotated for the proximal locking screw placement.

Anterior exposure to the glenohumeral joint for arthroplasty or glenoid fixation involves a lesser tuberosity osteotomy or subscapularis tenotomy. The capsule can remain with the subscapularis or can be separately mobilized depending on the procedure. The reapproximation of the subscapularis begins with reapproximation of the rotator interval and then proceeds with tendon-to-tendon sutures or with sutures from the bone to the tendon. The lesser tuberosity osteotomy[1] begins adjacent to the biceps groove and extends to the edge of the articular surface (**Fig. 5**A-F).

LATERAL OR ANTEROLATERAL APPROACH

This approach was developed as a method of more direct visualization of the greater tuberosity fragments and to mitigate the deltoid retraction issues. Whereas the deltopectoral exposure is truly an internervous dissection between the entire axillary nerve and the branches of the middle trunk, this approach is between axillary nerve branches to the middle and anterior deltoid. It can be considered a careful extension of the proximal exposure used for open rotator cuff repair.

Sequence of Steps for Dissection
• Proximal exposure (5 cm; **Figs. 6** and **7**)

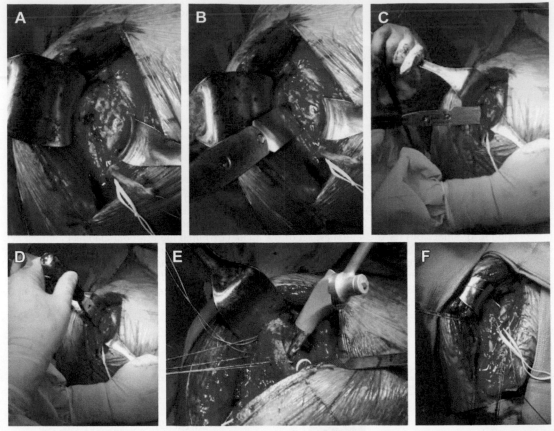

Fig. 5. (*A*) Lesser tuberosity osteotomy preparation. The biceps is removed from the bicepital groove and the medial border is further identified. (*B*) Before making the main cut, score the inferior aspect of the tuberosity with the chisel; use a sharp, disposable chisel. Then rotate arm to make a nice 2- to 4-mm-thick piece of lesser tuberosity. (*C, D*) Ensure that the osteotomy chisel is angled inferiorly and superiorly to create a clean cut. (*E*) Three #2 or #5 nonabsorbable sutures are used. The sutures can go from hole to hole in the superior to inferior or lateral to medial direction. (*F*) The medial to lateral sutures are used to cerclage the tuberosity and the superior to inferior lateral suture is used as a lateral based figure of 8 tension band.

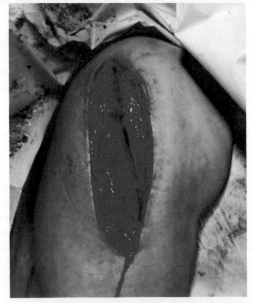

Fig. 6. Superficial dissection of the direct lateral or anterolateral approach. It is important to follow the fibers to the deltoid insertion.

- Find the anterior-middle deltoid raphe at the anterolateral corner of the acromion.
- Open the subacromial space and excise the bursa to expose to the greater tuberosity.
- Distal exposure (deltoid insertion, 10 cm)
  - Perform this part after the proximal exposure to expose the deltoid insertion.
  - It is important to divide the distal muscle fibers near the tendon insertion in line with the fibers that were divided proximally. This ensures that the muscle split will remain intact as the proximal and distal exposures are connected.
  - Elevate a portion of the anterior deltoid insertion to center the exposure for distal plate placement.
  - Middle exposure (at the level of the axillary nerve and usually at the inferior greater tuberosity fracture spike [**Fig. 8**]).
  - Connect the exposures by staying deep along the lateral humeral cortex.
  - This enables the surgeon to palpate the axillary nerve and branches from beneath.

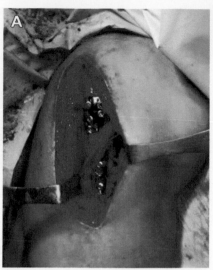
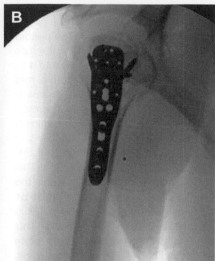

Fig. 7. (*A*) After completing the distal tendon dissection and elevation, the axillary nerve is maintained with the vascular pedicle and some adventitial fibers. The nerve is elevated from the periosteum and fracture so that the plate can be slid underneath the nerve. (*B*) The lateral radiograph of fixation with a location of the plate.

- Sweep the nerve away from the fracture and the perisoteum. The nerve can be quite adherent to the bone.
- This helps to further identify the nerve and its vascular pedicle. Keep the pedicle and surrounding soft tissue together.
- Finally, finish the deltoid split down to the already mobilized nerve. A few fibers can be also maintained with the nerve. During fracture fixation, the calcar screw holes are adjacent to the axillary nerve pedicle. Careful retraction of the pedicle is necessary for screw guide placement (**Fig. 9**).

MID HUMERUS AND EXTENSIONS FROM THE PROXIMAL APPROACHES

Both of the proximal humerus and shoulder exposures can be extended to the mid humerus. Similar to the proximal exposure, the muscle dissection is initially anterior. Then the musculature, in this case the brachialis, is retracted laterally for plate application.

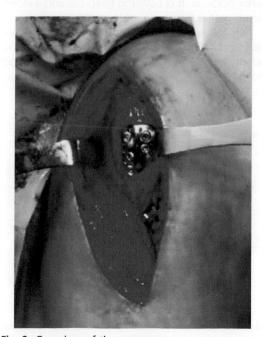

Fig. 8. By externally rotating the arm and humerus, the fracture can be reduced and the anteroposterior images can be obtained. This exposure permits easy handling.

Fig. 9. Overview of the exposure.

The incision is extended along the anterolateral arm such that, after the biceps fascia is incised, the muscle can be medially retracted. The deltoid fibers are elevated from the humerus for fracture reduction and plate application (**Figs. 10** and **11**). The brachialis is then readily evident for a mid muscle fiber split (**Fig. 12**). Although this exposure can be considered an internervous plane, the musculocutaneous nerve provides the prominent innervation (see **Fig. 12**). Divide the brachialis in a slightly more lateral position in an effort to maintain the distal musculocutaneous innervation. This can also facilitate radial nerve exposure within the brachialis muscle. The brachialis fibers must be fully elevated from the lateral cortex so that the radial nerve is mobilized with the brachialis. This helps to ensure that the laterally based plate does not pull the radial nerve from its anatomic position.[2]

If the fracture extends more proximally, the deltoid needs to be elevated in an appropriate manner so that the plate is perfectly centered on the proximal humerus shaft (**Fig. 13**). Because the humerus can be slightly bowed, if the plate is placed off center, the distal plate position can be really effected.

If the exposure was begun in the mid humerus and then extended proximally, the most common error is not to begin the elevation of the deltoid insertion elevation anterior enough. If the surgeon begins the deltoid insertion in the mid tendon rather than along the most anterior edge, then the deltoid needs to be split into anterior and posterior portions. It is better to keep the entire insertion together from anterior to posterior.

Rarely does the pectoralis insertion require division and in fact it provides excellent medial blood supply for the more proximal shaft/neck combined fractures.

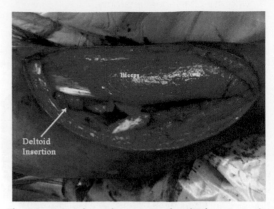

Fig. 11. Anterolateral extension for the humerus, the gunshot wound injury to the humerus is seen. The biceps in the central portion of the exposure. The deltoid insertion has been partially elevated.

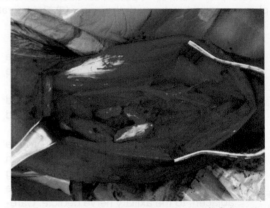

Fig. 12. The biceps is retracted in the medial direction with musculocutaneous nerve well visualized.

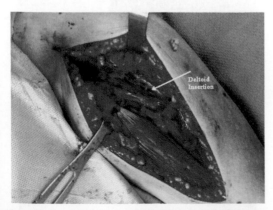

Fig. 10. A slightly more proximal left humerus fracture.

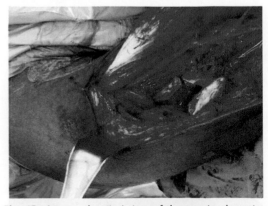

Fig. 13. A more detailed view of the proximal portion of the exposure in which the deltoid is elevated from the proximal fragment. Nearly the entire anterior portion must be elevated to place the plate in a lateral position.

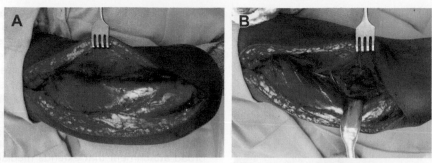

Fig. 14. (*A*) Posterior exposure of the entire humerus. The initial exposure involves identification of the lateral head of the triceps. (*B*) The distal lateral head of the triceps is elevated the supracondylar ridge. The posterior cutaneous branch of the radial nerve follows along the ridge.

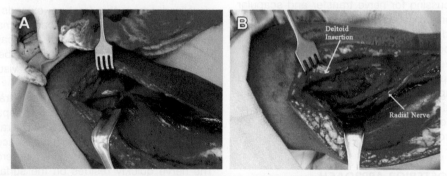

Fig. 15. (*A*) The proximal exposure involves elevation of the lateral triceps origin just distal to the deltoid insertion. (*B*) Posterior approach with the lateral triceps elevated in the medial direction. Radial nerve crosses in the midpoint of the humerus.

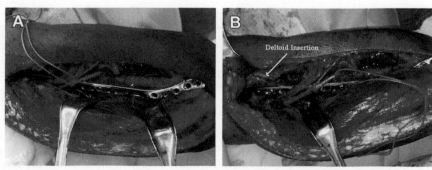

Fig. 16. (*A*) Distal aspect of the plate. The radial nerve is crossing in the midportion of the plate. (*B*) Proximal aspect of the plate.

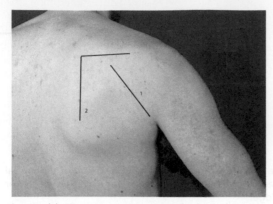

Fig. 17. (1) Direct posterior approach along the posterior deltoid. (2) Extensile Judet approach.

POSTERIOR SHOULDER AND UPPER APPROACH

Although this exposure is used infrequently, it is worth discussing for nerve transfer and scapular stabilization procedures.[3] These approaches are considered posterior in reference to the deltoid posterior border; thus, the superficial dissection involves developing this interval. The options include a direct approach to the posterior shoulder and lateral scapula, which utilizes the existing muscle planes and more extended approach to the scapula in which the posterior scapular muscles are elevated from medial to lateral.

DIRECT POSTERIOR APPROACH

Exposure for the axillary nerve (for triceps fascicular nerve transfer) and the glenohumeral joint involves mobilization or separation of the infraspinatus, teres minor, teres major, and latissimus tendons, and the myotendinous junctions. The authors prefer an incision nearly in line with the posterior deltoid for the proximal portion and then extended in between the lateral and long triceps heads as necessary

(Fig. 14). For proximal dissection, once the investing fascia of the deltoid is incised and the deltoid is retracted laterally, the infraspinatus is visualized bulging up from the scapula. The glenohumeral capsule and lateral scapula are visualized by finding the interval between the infraspinatus and teres minor more medially and then extending laterally toward the joint (Fig. 15). This is a true internervous plane between the suprascapular nerve and a direct teres minor nerve branch. The joint capsule has a broad attachment that extends medially from the glenoid rim to the scapular neck. To gain access to the glenoid humeral joint rather than the lateral scapula, use a needle to find the joint as a location for capsulotomy because it is quite lateral (Fig. 16).

Another helpful landmark is that the teres minor has a much thinner muscle body than the broad infraspinatus muscle. By mobilizing the muscle units, the exposure to the scapula can be efficient for most scapular neck and some body fractures. If the medial scapula or vertebral portion needs to visualized when the fracture extends into the spine, then a counterincision can be made along the superior medial portion of the scapula. The medial infraspinatus muscle belly can be elevated easily from the superior angle to visualize the fracture.[4]

For a triceps motor to axillary nerve transfer, the dissection begins distally through separation of the lateral and long triceps heads. The radial nerve is seen exiting from the triangle space with its vascular pedicle just beneath the teres major. The nerve quickly resides on the surface of the deep triceps head and begins branching to the long head of triceps. Transfer of these branches is most ideal from a functional standpoint because the long head is also an arm adductor, and restoration of abduction is the goal. The authors have found that these branches are not as good from a microsurgical standpoint because they quickly arborize and there is a short turning distance toward the axillary nerve. Using electrical

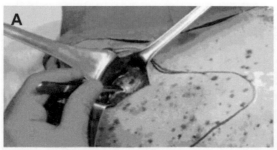
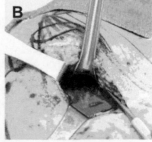

Fig. 18. (A, B) Direct posterior approach. (A) After elevation and retraction of the deltoid in the lateral direction, the infraspinatus is well visualized. (B) The interval between the infraspinatus and teres minor has been developed to expose the lateral edge of the scapula. (Photo Courtesy of Peter Cole, MD.)

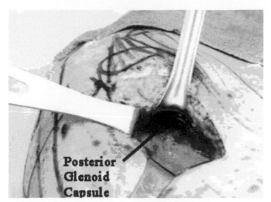

Fig. 19. Further retraction enables visualization of the posterior glenohumeral joint capsule. (*Photo Courtesy of* Peter Cole, MD.)

stimulation, 2 redundant branches to the lateral head provide a good size match to the anterior division of the axillary nerve and have effective length for a tension-free anastomosis.

If additional fracture fixation in this middle to upper humerus is necessary during the nerve procedures, the surgeon must use an extension of the posterior exposure. The triceps can be split along the natural plane between the lateral and long heads, or can be mobilized as an entire unit from lateral to medial. This latter approach is an extension of the posterolateral or posterior approaches for the mid to distal humerus (addressed by Capo, Criner, and Shamian elsewhere in this issue; **Figs. 17–19**).

EXTENSILE (JUDET) APPROACH

This exposure is indicated for scapular body fractures that are multifragmentary.[5] It involves elevating the muscle innervated by the suprascapular nerve (infraspinatus and supraspinatus) from its scapular origins. It can be difficult to reach the inferior glenohumeral joint and inferior scapular margin.

The incision extends along the scapula in an L-shaped fashion with a liberal subcutaneous dissection to identify the infraspinatus. The muscle is elevated from the lateral and superior border just inferior to the scapular spine. When the exposure reaches the lateral border, care is taken around the spinal glenoid notch because the nerve can be placed on tension by the fracture and retraction (**Fig. 20**).

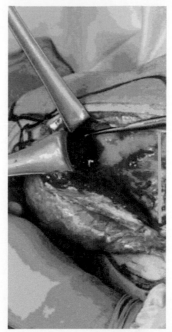

Fig. 20. Judet approach. The infraspinatus and teres minor have been elevated from their origin (*colored line*). The hook is around the suprascapular nerve as it crosses in the spinal glenoid notch. The entire scapular body can be seen. (*Photo Courtesy of* Peter Cole, MD.)

REFERENCES

1. Lapner PL, Sabri E, Rakhra K, et al. Comparison of lesser tuberosity osteotomy to subscapularis peel in shoulder arthroplasty: a randomized controlled trial. J Bone Joint Surg Am 2012; 94(24):2239–46.

2. McKee MD, Kim J, Kebaish K, et al. Functional outcome after open supracondylar fractures of the humerus. The effect of the surgical approach. J Bone Joint Surg Br 2000;82(5):646–51.

3. Zlotolow DA, Catalano LW III, Barron OA, et al. Surgical exposures of the humerus. J Am Acad Orthop Surg 2006;14:754–65.

4. Gauger EM, Cole PA. Surgical technique: a minimally invasive approach to scapula neck and body fractures. Clin Orthop Relat Res 2011;469(12): 3390–9.

5. Jones CB, Cornelius JP, Sietsema DL, et al. Modified Judet approach and minifragment fixation of scapular body and glenoid neck fractures. J Orthop Trauma 2009;23(8):558–64.

Exposures of the Humerus for Fracture Fixation

John T. Capo, MD[a],*, Katharine T. Criner, MD[b], Ben Shamian, MD[c]

KEYWORDS

- Humerus • Fracture • Radial nerve • Exposure

KEY POINTS

- Most humerus fractures can be treated closed and most radial nerve injuries spontaneously recover.
- Plating of humeral shaft fractures results in reliable healing and good functional results.
- Midshaft fractures of the humerus can be plated from an anterior, posterior, or posterolateral approach.
- Intramedullary fixation of the humerus gives less reliable results than plating.
- Posterior exposures of the upper arm must respect and protect the triceps mechanism and ulnar nerve.

ANATOMY OF THE ARM

The humerus is the largest bone in the upper limb. It articulates with the scapula at the glenohumeral joint proximally and at the radius and the ulna distally at the elbow joint. The 3 zones of the humerus are the proximal humerus, the humeral shaft, and the distal humerus. The proximal humerus consists of 4 parts: the articular head, lesser tuberosity, greater tuberosity, and proximal metaphysis and shaft. The hemispherical head articulates with the glenoid cavity of the scapula. The junction of the articular portion and the remaining head is called the anatomic neck, whereas the junction between the head fragment and the shaft, below the tuberosities, is termed the surgical neck. The surgical neck is the most common site of proximal humerus fractures. The axillary nerve and posterior circumflex humeral vessels travel along the posterior aspect of the surgical neck.

The greater tuberosity is located lateral to the bicipital groove. It is the point of attachment of 3 rotator cuff muscles: the supraspinatus, infraspinatus, and the teres minor. The suprascapular nerve innervates the supraspinatus and infraspinatus. The axillary nerve innervates the teres minor. The lesser tuberosity is located medial to the bicipital groove and is the site of subscapularis insertion. The subscapularis is innervated by the upper and lower subscapular nerves.

The shaft of the humerus is tubular and has 2 important prominent features: the deltoid tuberosity laterally and the spiral groove posteriorly. The deltoid muscle inserts on the deltoid tuberosity and is innervated by the axillary nerve. The radial nerve and deep brachial artery run in the spiral groove.[1]

The distal humerus fans out into 2 columns and supports the elbow articular surface. The elbow joint consists of the spooled trochlea (articulating

Disclosure: K.T. Criner, MD, and B. Shamian, MD, have nothing to disclose. J.T. Capo, MD, is a paid consultant for DePuy-Synthes. Some of the case examples have plates manufactured by this company, but no direct financial relationship exists in relation to this work.

[a] Department of Orthopaedics, NYU Langone Medical Center, NYU Hospital for Joint Diseases, 530 First Avenue, Suite 8U, New York, NY 10016, USA; [b] Division of Hand Surgery, Department of Orthopaedics, NYU Hospital for Joint Diseases, 550 First Avenue, Suite 8U, New York, NY 10016, USA; [c] Department of Medicine, NYU Woodhull Medical Center, 760 Broadway, Brooklyn, NY 11206, USA

* Corresponding author.

E-mail address: john.capo@nyumc.org

hand.theclinics.com

with the ulna distally and medially); the capitellum (articulating with the radial head distally and laterally); and 3 fossae (radial fossa and coronoid fossa anteriorly, and olecranon fossa posteriorly). Certain areas of the humerus are clinically important because they are in direct contact with the indicated nerves:

- Surgical neck: axillary nerve
- Spiral groove: radial nerve
- Medial epicondyle: ulnar nerve posterior to it
- Lateral epicondyle: radial nerve anterior to it

The arm consists of 2 compartments: the anterior or flexor compartment and the posterior or extensor compartment. The anterior compartment contains 3 flexor muscles, which are all innervated by the musculocutaneous nerve (**Fig. 1**). The biceps brachii has a short head and a long head, each with different sites of origin. The short head originates from the coracoid process of the scapula and the long head originates from the supraglenoid tubercle of the scapula. The biceps muscle terminates distally into 1 tendon and a fascial

extension. The biceps tendon attaches to the ulnar side of the bicipital tuberosity on the radius. The fascial bicipital aponeurosis, also known as the lacertus fibrosis, fans onto the ulnar part of the antebrachial fascia and medial epicondyle. The blood supply of the biceps brachii is via the brachial artery. The biceps flexes and supinates the forearm at the elbow.

The brachialis muscle originates from the lower half of the anterior surface of the humerus and inserts distally on to the coronoid process of the ulna (**Fig. 2**). The brachialis is the main flexor of the elbow. The brachial artery and radial recurrent artery are the blood supply to the brachialis muscle. The brachial artery and median, ulnar, and musculocutaneous nerves course medial to the brachialis and biceps muscles (**Fig. 3**).

The coracobrachialis originates from the apex of the coracoid process of the scapula and it inserts on the middle and medial surface of the humerus. The coracobrachialis and the short head of the biceps brachii form the conjoined tendon. The coracobrachialis is the smallest of the 3 muscles

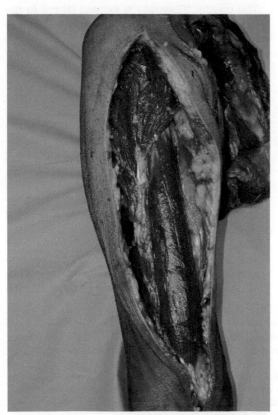

Fig. 1. Anterior compartment of the arm showing the deltoid muscle proximally and the biceps and brachialis muscles distally. (*Courtesy of* **J.T. Capo, MD,** New York, NY. Copyright © 2014. All Rights Reserved.)

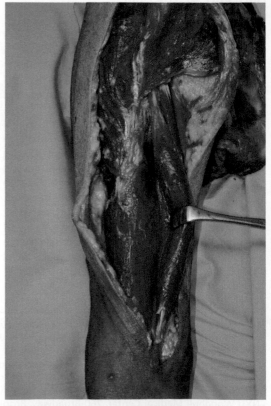

Fig. 2. The biceps muscle is retracted medially to show the underlying brachialis muscle, which covers the anterior humeral shaft. (*Courtesy of* **J.T. Capo, MD,** New York, NY. Copyright © 2014. All Rights Reserved.)

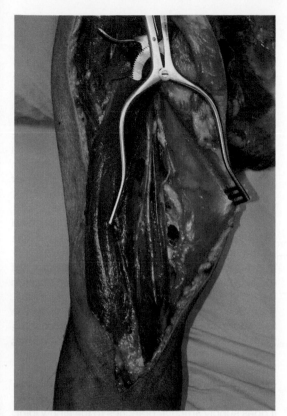

Fig. 3. The biceps and brachialis muscles are retracted laterally exposing the brachial artery and vein, as well as the median and ulnar nerves. (*Courtesy of* J.T. Capo, MD, New York, NY. Copyright © 2014. All Rights Reserved.)

(coracobrachialis, short head of biceps, and pectoralis minor) that originate from the coracoid process. The coracobrachialis inserts between the origins of the brachialis and triceps brachii. This muscle has 2 important anatomic landmarks. The musculocutaneous nerve pierces the muscle 5 to 6 cm from its origin. Its distal insertion indicates the location of the nutrient foramen of the humerus, where the main nutrient artery penetrates the bone, and the location where the ulnar nerve courses from anterior to posterior and penetrates the intermuscular septum.[1] The coracobrachialis receives blood supply from the brachial artery. The coracobrachialis flexes and adducts the shoulder. It also internally rotates the shoulder.

The posterior compartment contents include 2 extensor muscles innervated by the radial nerve. The triceps brachii comprises a medial (or short) head, a long head, and a lateral head. The long head originates from the infraglenoid tuberosity of the scapula, the lateral head (strongest) originates from the superior half of the posterior-lateral

surface of the humerus, and the medial head originates from the inferior two-thirds of the posterior surface of the humerus, beginning at the spiral groove (**Fig. 4**). The medial head surrounds the radial nerve in the spiral groove. The 3 heads converge to form 1 tendon, which inserts on the proximal end of the ulna at the olecranon process. Its blood supply is the profunda brachii artery of the arm. The triceps brachii extends the forearm at the elbow. The long head also provides adduction and extension of the arm at the shoulder.

The anconeus is a small, triangular muscle that originates from the posterior surface of the lateral epicondyle of the humerus. It inserts on the lateral surface of the olecranon process and posterior surface of the proximal ulna. The radial nerve innervates the anconeus, which provides extension and pronation of the forearm at the elbow. The anconeus receives blood supply from the interosseous recurrent artery.

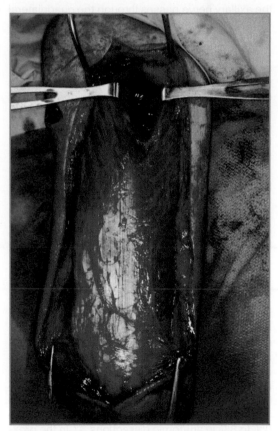

Fig. 4. The posterior aspect of the arm is visualized with the 3 heads of the triceps muscle joining distally at the common triceps tendon. The long and lateral heads are split proximally to visualize the radial nerve and profunda brachii artery. (*Courtesy of* J.T. Capo, MD, New York, NY. Copyright © 2014. All Rights Reserved.)

NERVES OF THE ARM

There are 5 main peripheral nerves that travel in the arm: axillary, median, ulnar, musculocutaneous, and radial nerves. Most of the nerves and arteries in the arm are on the medial aspect of the anterior compartment.

AXILLARY NERVE (C5, C6)

The axillary nerve develops from the posterior cord of the brachial plexus and then travels behind the axillary artery at the level of the axilla. It runs anterior on the inferolateral surface of the subscapularis, 3 to 5 mm medial to the musculotendinous border.[2] The axillary nerve then travels along the inferior border of the shoulder capsule and then through the quadrangular space with the posterior humeral circumflex artery and vein below the lower border of the teres minor. The quadrangular space is formed by the humerus laterally, long head of the triceps medially, teres major inferiorly, and teres minor superiorly. After the axillary nerve passes through the quadrilateral space, at the inferior border of the subscapularis muscle and posterior border of the humerus neck, it divides into its terminal branches.[3] The anterior trunk branch wraps around the surgical neck of the humerus on the undersurface of the deltoid and supplies the middle and anterior deltoid. The anterior branch terminates in small cutaneous branches that provide sensation to the anterolateral shoulder. The posterior branch supplies the teres minor muscle and posterior part of the deltoid muscle. The posterior branch pierces the deep fascia and terminates as the superior lateral cutaneous nerve of the arm, which provides sensation to the lateral shoulder. The articular branch enters the shoulder joint inferior to the subscapularis.[3]

MUSCULOCUTANEOUS NERVE (C5, C6)

The musculocutaneous nerve arises from the lateral cord of the brachial plexus. Its proximal location is lateral to the median nerve. As it descends to the arm, it pierces the coracobrachialis approximately 5 to 8 cm distal to the coracoid[4] and supplies motor innervation to the coracobrachialis. The prevalence of cases of the musculocutaneous nerve located outside (not piercing) the coracobrachialis muscle is reported to be 0% to 8% in anatomic dissections.[5–7] In the proximal third of the arm, it is located between the biceps brachii and the brachialis and gives motor innervation to these muscles. The musculocutaneous nerve then pierces the deep fascia lateral to the biceps brachii at the level just above the elbow. The nerve then emerges lateral to the distal biceps tendon and brachioradialis to terminate as the lateral antebrachial cutaneous nerve, which innervates the radial side of the forearm. Variation exists with regard to communication between the musculocutaneous nerve and the median nerve. In an anatomic dissection of 56 upper limbs, communications were seen between the musculocutaneous and median nerves in 53.6% of the arms.[8]

MEDIAN NERVE IN THE ARM (C6, C7, C8, T1)

The median nerve arises from the medial and lateral cords of the brachial plexus. The median nerve runs lateral to the brachial artery on top of the coracobrachialis muscle until it reaches the middle of the arm, where it crosses to the medial side and passes over the brachialis muscle. It runs along the medial edge of the biceps brachii, with the brachial artery lying lateral to it. In the antecubital fossa, the median nerve lies deep to the bicipital aponeurosis (lacertus fibrosis) medial to the antecubital vein, the brachial artery, and the biceps tendon, and lateral to the common origin of the flexor and pronator muscles.[4] The median nerve has no branches in the arm, but it does supply articular branches to the elbow joint. The median nerve may become entrapped at 5 potential sites: supracondylar process, ligament of Struthers, lacertus fibrosis, between the ulnar and humeral heads of the pronator teres, and the flexor digitorum superficialis aponeurotic arch. The supracondylar process is a residual osseous structure on the distal humerus that is present in 1% of the population. The ligament of Struthers is an abnormal fibrous band structure that originates 5 cm proximal to the medial epicondyle at the tip of the supracondylar process and runs distally to insert on the medial epicondyle.[4] The lacertus fibrosis is a normal fascial sleeve that extends from the biceps tendon to the medial epicondyle and covers the median nerve and brachial artery. In relation to the brachial artery, the median nerve is lateral to it in the upper part, anterior in the middle part, and medial to the artery in the lower arm. The median nerve enters the forearm between the pronator teres and biceps tendon, then travels between the flexor digitorum superficialis (FDS) and flexor digitorum profundus, and typically lies under the FDS to the middle finger. The median nerve then emerges between the FDS and flexor pollicis longus. The terminal branches of the median nerve are the anterior interosseous branch, palmar cutaneous branch, recurrent motor branch, and digital cutaneous branches.

ULNAR NERVE IN THE ARM (C8, T1)

The ulnar nerve arises from the medial cord of the brachial plexus and runs posteromedial to the brachial artery. It descends proximally medial to the coracobrachialis and anterior to the long head of the triceps. In the middle of the arm, at the level of the distal attachment of the coracobrachialis to the humerus, together with the superior ulnar collateral artery and its venae comitantes, the nerve pierces the medial intermuscular septum at the arcade of Struthers to enter the posterior compartment of the brachium.[4] This point has been found to average 10 cm proximal to the medial epicondyle.[9] The ulnar nerve distally passes medial and posterior to the medial epicondyle of the humerus and lateral to the olecranon process in the cubital tunnel. In this area the nerve is superficial, easily palpable, and vulnerable to injury. Like the median nerve, the ulnar nerve has no branches in the arm, but it also supplies articular proprioception branches to the elbow joint. The ulnar nerve then enters the forearm between the 2 heads (humeral and ulnar) of the flexor carpi ulnaris and courses between the flexor carpi ulnaris and flexor digitorum profundus muscles.

The ulnar nerve has several possible compression sites as it courses from proximal to distal: the medial intermuscular septum, arcade of Struthers, medial epicondyle, Osborne ligament, anconeus epitrochlearis, aponeurosis of the 2 heads of the flexor carpi ulnaris, and the deep flexor/pronator aponeurosis. The arcade of Struthers is an area of transverse fascial fibers that connect the medial head of the triceps to the intermuscular septum approximately 8 to 10 cm proximal to the medial epicondyle.[10] The thickness of these fibers is variable among patients. A true arcade is found in approximately 60% to 70% of the population.[11] The arcade of Struthers is much more common than the ligament of Struthers (median nerve entrapment), which is found in 1% of the population.[12] The medial epicondyle could have osteophytes causing compression of the ulnar nerve. The Osborne ligament is the cubital tunnel retinaculum, which serves as the roof of the cubital tunnel. The posterior and transverse bands of the medial collateral ligament serve as the floor of the cubital tunnel. The anconeus epitrochlearis muscle is an anomalous muscle that replaces the Osborne ligament in 11% of the population.

RADIAL NERVE IN THE ARM (C5, C6, C7, C8, T1)

The radial nerve, arising from the posterior cord of the brachial plexus, supplies all the muscles in the posterior compartment of the arm and forearm.

The radial nerve courses on the posterior wall of the axilla, posterior to the brachial artery, medial to the humerus, and anterior to the long head of the triceps. It gives branches that innervate the long and the medial heads of triceps brachii and posterior cutaneous nerve of the arm before it crosses the humerus. The radial nerve then passes through the triangular interval with the profunda brachii artery in the posterior compartment between the long head of triceps and humerus (**Fig. 5**). Next the radial nerve travels around the humeral shaft in the spiral groove with the deep brachial artery of the arm in direct contact with the humeral shaft. Along the spiral groove the radial nerve gives branches to the inferior lateral cutaneous nerve of the arm, posterior cutaneous nerve of the forearm, lateral head of the triceps, medial head of triceps, and anconeus. After crossing the humerus, it pierces the lateral intermuscular septum approximately 10 to 12 cm from the lateral epicondyle coursing from the posterior to anterior compartments.[13–15] This point is between the deltoid insertion and the brachialis origin. It then runs

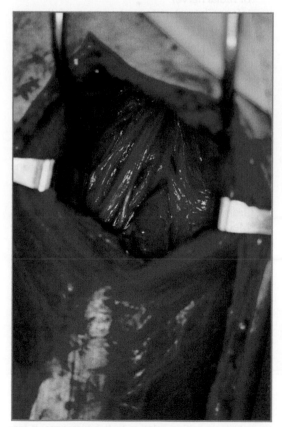

Fig. 5. The radial nerve and deep brachial artery are seen deep to the triceps muscle lying on the posterior humeral shaft. (*Courtesy of* J.T. Capo, MD, New York, NY. Copyright © 2014. All Rights Reserved.)

between the brachialis and brachioradialis to lie anterior to the lateral epicondyle of the humerus. One to 3 cm distal to the lateral epicondyle and deep to the brachioradialis, the radial nerve splits into the superficial sensory branch of the radial nerve and the posterior interosseous nerve.[16,17]

Among the major nerves in the upper extremity, radial nerve entrapment is the least common. Radial nerve palsy in the arm most commonly is caused by fractures of the humerus, especially in the middle third (Holstein-Lewis fracture). It can also be compressed by the lateral intermuscular septum. Although rare, an anomalous muscle, the accessory subscapularis-teres-latissimus, has been reported to cause compression of the radial nerve at this level.[18]

CUTANEOUS INNERVATIONS OF THE ARM

Posterior surface of the arm:

- Superior lateral cutaneous nerve of the arm (branch of axillary nerve)
- Posterior cutaneous nerve of the arm (branch of radial nerve)
- Inferior lateral cutaneous nerve of the arm (branch of radial nerve)

Lateral surface of the arm:

- Superior lateral cutaneous nerve of the arm (branch of axillary nerve)
- Inferior lateral cutaneous nerve of the arm (branch of radial nerve)

Medial surface of the arm:

- Intercostobrachial nerve (lateral cutaneous branch of T2)
- Medial brachial cutaneous nerve of the arm (from medial cord of brachial plexus)
- Medial antebrachial cutaneous nerve of the arm (from medial cord of brachial plexus)

ARTERIES OF THE ARM
The Brachial Artery

The teres major marks the end of the axillary artery and beginning of the brachial artery. During its course through the arm, the brachial artery lies anterior to the triceps brachii and brachialis muscles, and is overlapped by the biceps brachii and coracobrachialis muscles. The artery lies medial to the humerus proximally. As it descends, accompanying the median nerve, the artery is located in an anterior position relative to the humerus. It terminates in the cubital fossa under the bicipital aponeurosis, dividing into the 2 major arteries of the forearm, the radial and ulnar arteries, at the

level of the neck of the radius. Major branches in the arm are the deep brachial artery of the arm (profunda brachii artery), the superior ulnar collateral artery, the inferior ulnar collateral artery, and the nutrient humeral artery. The profunda brachii artery travels with the radial nerve and is the largest branch of the brachial artery. The superior ulnar collateral artery arises from the brachial artery and accompanies the ulnar nerve, piercing the medial intermuscular septum to end proximally, posterior to the medial epicondyle of the humerus. The ulnar artery gives rise to both the anterior ulnar recurrent artery, which joins the inferior ulnar collateral anterior to the medial epicondyle of the humerus, and the posterior ulnar recurrent artery, which joins the superior ulnar collateral artery posterior to the medial humeral epicondyle.[19,20] The radial artery gives off the radial recurrent artery, which joins with the radial recurrent branch of the deep artery of the arm anterior to the lateral epicondyle.

SUPERFICIAL VEINS OF THE ARM

The veins of the arm are divided into superficial and deep. The two systems frequently anastomose. The superficial veins are located immediately beneath the skin. The deep veins accompany the arteries. The 2 main superficial veins are the basilic and the cephalic veins. The basilic vein, visible through the skin, runs on the medial aspect of the arm. It ascends in the groove between the biceps brachii and pronator teres. It perforates the deep fascia, running on the medial side of the brachial artery. It finally drains into the axillary vein. The cephalic vein ascends on the lateral side of the arm in front of the elbow in the groove between the brachioradialis and the biceps brachii. It continues up in the deltopectoral groove, piercing the clavipectoral fascia to drain into the axillary vein.

SUMMARY

The anterior (flexor) compartment contents include:

- The flexor muscles: coracobrachialis, biceps brachii, and brachialis
- The brachial artery and branches
- The median nerve
- The ulnar nerve (proximally)
- The musculocutaneous nerve
- The basilic vein

The posterior (extensor) compartment contents include:

- The extensor muscles (triceps)
- The radial nerve and branches

- The profunda brachii artery
- The ulnar nerve (distally)

SURGICAL APPROACHES

Various approaches to the humerus have been described: the anterior approach, the anterolateral approach, the posterior triceps-splitting approach, the posterior paratricipital approach, and the extended posterior-lateral exposure. The radial nerve is at greatest risk during exposure of the humeral shaft in the posterior and lateral approaches.

ANTERIOR APPROACH TO THE HUMERUS

The patient is positioned supine with a bump under the scapula. The operative arm is placed abducted approximately 45° on a hand table during this approach. The incision is made longitudinally from the tip of the coracoid process distally in line with the deltopectoral groove and continued along the lateral aspect of the biceps muscle and tendon. The incision stops 3 cm proximal to the anterior elbow flexion crease. The incision may be shortened and centered on the level of the fracture if used for fracture fixation. The deep dissection proximally is between the deltoid (axillary nerve) laterally and the biceps (musculocutaneous nerve) medially. The distal dissection involves splitting the brachialis muscle between its lateral and medial portions (**Fig. 6**). This plane is internervous. The musculocutaneous nerve innervates the medial side of the brachialis and the radial nerve innervates the lateral aspect. At-risk structures during the distal dissection are the radial nerve as it runs between the brachialis and brachioradialis. The lateral antebrachial cutaneous nerve is at risk as it travels between the brachialis and biceps. The exposure allows access proximally from the humeral head to the coronoid fossa distally. Indications for the anterior approach include the following[3]:

- Anterior plating of fractures of the proximal and middle thirds of the humerus
- Osteotomy of the humerus
- Biopsy and resection of bone tumors
- Treatment of osteomyelitis
- Extension of deltopectoral approach

This approach allows access and repair of fractures of the humeral shaft from the humeral neck, to midshaft, and down to the distal third of the shaft. Fractures of the middle third to the midshaft may be stabilized by a 4.5-mm or 3.5-mm dynamic compression plate (**Fig. 7**). The proximal extension of this approach allows fixation into the humeral head and down into the humeral shaft for fractures of the humeral neck with shaft extension (**Fig. 8**).

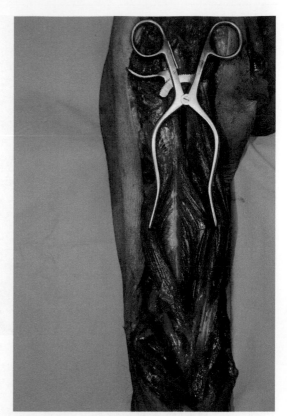

Fig. 6. The anterior approach to the humerus requires medial retraction of the biceps brachii and then central splitting of the underlying brachialis muscle. This is an internervous plane because the brachialis is innervated by the radial nerve laterally and the musculocutaneous nerve medially. (*Courtesy of* J.T. Capo, MD, New York, NY. Copyright © 2014. All Rights Reserved.)

ANTEROLATERAL APPROACH TO THE HUMERUS

The patient is positioned supine with a bump under the scapula. The operative arm is placed at the patient's side on a hand table. The anterolateral approach begins with a curved longitudinal incision over the lateral border of the biceps, starting about 10 cm proximal to the flexion crease of the elbow and extending to the lateral epicondyle. The deep interval is between the brachialis and the brachioradialis. The radial nerve is located in this interval between the brachialis and brachioradialis and courses from posterior to anterior. The approach exposes the distal fourth of the humerus and distally to the lateral epicondyle.[21] Through this interval the radial nerve can be traced from the midhumerus to the proximal forearm. Care must be taken distally not to injure the lateral antebrachial cutaneous nerve as it exits between the biceps and brachialis muscles. The radial nerve

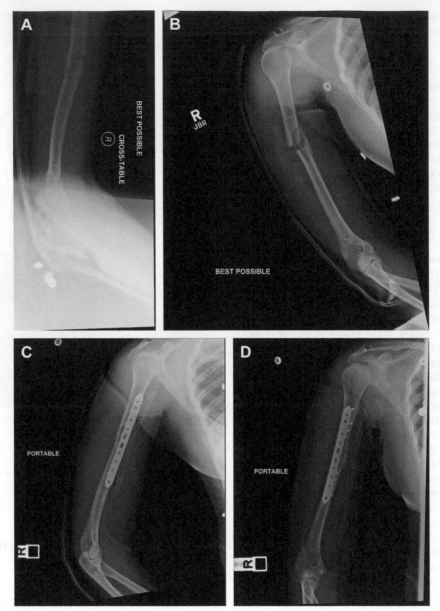

Fig. 7. (*A, B*) Anteroposterior (AP) and lateral views showing a comminuted proximal third right humeral shaft fracture in a 37-year-old patient with poly trauma, who also sustained a left scapula and clavicle fracture. (*C, D*) AP and lateral postoperative views showing stable fixation with a 3.5-mm dynamic compression plate using a combination of locking and nonlocking screws. (*Courtesy of* J.T. Capo, MD, New York, NY. Copyright © 2014. All Rights Reserved.)

is likewise at risk from distal extension and must be identified between the brachialis and brachioradialis at the lateral epicondyle.[21] Indications for the anterolateral approach are exposure of the anterior to middle one-third of the humerus.

POSTERIOR APPROACHES TO THE HUMERUS

The patient is positioned in the lateral decubitus position with the arm over a bolster. The surgical

incision is longitudinal in the midline of the posterior aspect of the arm, from 8 cm below the acromion to the olecranon fossa. The incision should gently curve radially around the olecranon process, to avoid an incision directly over the bony prominence of the olecranon (**Fig. 9**). The superficial dissection involves mobilizing lateral and medial flaps. The ulnar nerve is at risk during the medial flap exposure and should be mobilized and protected if needed.

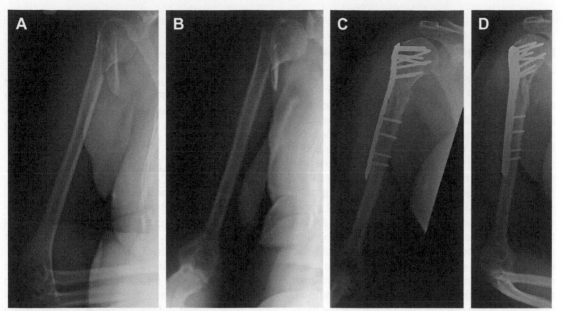

Fig. 8. (*A, B*) Shoulder and humerus films in a 54-year-old man who was in a motorcycle accident, showing a humeral neck fracture with extension into the shaft. (*C, D*) Postoperative radiographs showing fracture stabilization with a locking plate into the humeral head with plate extension onto the shaft. (*Courtesy of* F. Liporace, MD, New York, NY.)

The posterior approaches provide excellent access to the distal three-fourths of the posterior aspect of the humerus. The radial nerve is at risk during the posterior approaches as it runs in the spiral groove of the humerus. The posterior approaches vary in how the triceps muscle is mobilized. In all cases of exposure of the humerus through a posterior approach the ulnar nerve needs to be identified, mobilized, and protected during the dissection and, at times, transposed after fracture fixation.

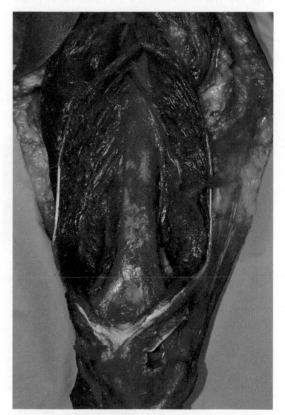

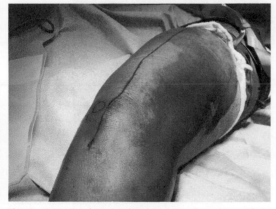

Fig. 9. Posterior longitudinal incision for approach to humeral shaft. The distal aspect is curved laterally to avoid the tip of the olecranon. This incision can be used for all of the various deep posterior approaches to the humeral shaft and distal humerus. (*Courtesy of* J.T. Capo, MD, New York, NY. Copyright © 2014. All Rights Reserved.)

Fig. 10. Posterior triceps-splitting approach to the humeral shaft and distal aspect. The radial nerve and deep brachial artery are seen proximally coursing from medial to lateral. The distal limit of this approach is the olecranon fossa. (*Courtesy of* J.T. Capo, MD, New York, NY. Copyright © 2014. All Rights Reserved.)

POSTERIOR TRICEPS-SPLITTING APPROACH

The deep dissection involves separating the 2 superficial heads of the triceps brachii muscle (the long and lateral heads). The interval is easier to palpate proximally, before they become the common tendon. The medial head of the triceps is located deep to the long and lateral heads and it originates from the distal-medial aspect of the spiral groove. The medial head is split down to the periosteum of the humeral shaft. The spiral groove contains the radial nerve; thus, the radial nerve separates the origins of the lateral and medial heads of the triceps. The radial nerve either lies directly on the bone or it lies on the medial head of the triceps. A reliable place to locate the radial nerve is approximately 2 finger breadths proximal to the most proximal aspect of the triceps tendon, described as the point of confluence.[22] If the muscle bellies are split in this location, the nerve can reliably be found lying on the posterior humerus. The humerus can be exposed from the proximal third to the olecranon fossa through this approach (Fig. 10). The limitations are the radial nerve proximally and the olecranon distally. It is difficult to explore an injured radial nerve fully through this approach.

The exposure can be extended distally by splitting the triceps tendon along the olecranon.[23] Through this extension, the medial and lateral columns and the proximal aspect of the articular surface can be exposed (Fig. 11A). Further exposure of the joint can be achieved through hyperflexion of the elbow and resection of the tip of the olecranon (see Fig. 11B). The distal aspect of the joint surface can be visualized well, but it is difficult to see the anterior aspect of the joint through the triceps-splitting approach.

PARATRICIPITAL APPROACH

The medial and lateral aspects of the triceps can be elevated from either or both sides of the humerus. The lateral exposure is between the lateral head of the triceps and the lateral intermuscular septum. Identification of the radial nerve is approximately 14 cm proximal to the lateral epicondyle and it pierces the lateral intermuscular septum 10 cm proximal to the articular surface. The posterior antebrachial cutaneous nerve courses along the posterior aspect of the lateral intermuscular septum and it can be traced proximally to where it branches off from the radial nerve as the radial nerve exits the spiral groove. In this approach, the radial nerve with the posterior cutaneous nerve is carefully mobilized from the humerus. The triceps muscle can then be subperiosteally elevated and retracted medially and the lateral column of the humeral shaft can be exposed (Fig. 12A). The ulnar nerve is at risk when the medial side is approached. The ulnar nerve must be identified on the medial column and traced proximally to

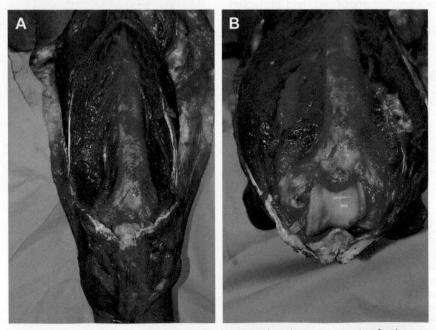

Fig. 11. (A) The triceps tendon can be split longitudinally onto the olecranon to give further exposure of the distal humerus. (B) Further splitting and hyperflexion of the joint allows improved visualization of the distal humeral articular surface. (*Courtesy of* J.T. Capo, MD, New York, NY. Copyright © 2014. All Rights Reserved.)

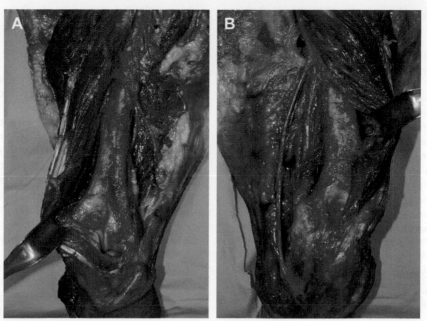

Fig. 12. (*A*) The triceps muscle is elevated off the posterior humerus with care taken to protect the radial nerve. The humeral shaft is exposed with extension down to the distal aspect of the lateral column. The radial head can be visualized distally. (*B*) The medial column of the humerus is visualized with lateral retraction of the triceps muscle. The ulnar nerve has been transposed anteriorly. (*Courtesy of* J.T. Capo, MD, New York, NY. Copyright © 2014. All Rights Reserved.)

the intermuscular septum and distally to the cubital tunnel. After the nerve is elevated and retracted, the triceps can be reflected from medial to lateral and the medial column of the humerus exposed (see **Fig. 12**B). The medial humeral shaft and medial humeral column are easily exposed through this exposure. This exposure is ideal for distal third humeral shaft and extra-articular supracondylar fractures. Simple intra-articular fractures of the distal humerus can be addressed using this approach. The joint surface can be visualized by hyperflexion of the elbow and retraction of the triceps with elbow extension.

EXTENDED POSTERIOR-LATERAL APPROACH

The superficial dissection begins with identifying the posterior antebrachial cutaneous nerve in the subcutaneous tissue and then on the posterior aspect of the lateral intermuscular septum, and tracing it proximally to the radial nerve proper. This nerve pattern can be inconsistent at times, and often the best dissection technique is to find the main radial nerve primarily. The radial nerve is followed to the level proximal to where it pierces the lateral intermuscular septum. The lateral intermuscular septum overlying the radial nerve is then released for several centimeters. The septum release aids in mobilization of the radial nerve. The lateral head of the triceps is subperiosteally reflected from lateral to medial, exposing the humeral shaft up to the level of the axillary nerve at the neck of the humerus and to the distal extent

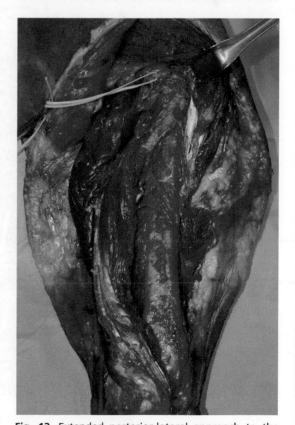

Fig. 13. Extended posterior-lateral approach to the humerus. The deltoid muscle is retracted proximally revealing the axillary nerve (in vessel loop). The interval above and below the radial nerve can be used. (*Courtesy of* J.T. Capo, MD, New York, NY. Copyright © 2014. All Rights Reserved.)

of the lateral column (**Fig. 13**). Approximately 94% of the humeral diaphysis can be exposed with this approach.[24] The entire radial nerve can be identified from the medial humerus to the radial tunnel. It is an excellent approach to plate the humeral diaphysis while exploring the radial nerve. Fixation of the humerus can be accomplished from the proximal third to the lateral column distally all the way to the posterior aspect of the capitellum (**Fig. 14**). The profunda brachii artery runs with the radial nerve in the spiral groove and must also be protected. The distal 55% of the humeral shaft can be exposed if the radial nerve is not mobilized.[24] The humeral shaft can be exposed proximal to the nerve up to the proximal third of the humerus and distal to the nerve to the olecranon fossa, and down to the posterior aspect of the capitellum.

PEARLS AND PITFALLS

- Any posterior exposure of the arm first demands identification and protection of the ulnar nerve.
- The ulnar nerve needs to be mobilized and protected in all cases of fixation of the humeral medial column, but transposition is only necessary if the nerve impinges on the plate.
- The extended posterior-lateral approach (EPLA) is the most versatile exposure to simultaneously stabilize a humeral shaft fracture and explore the radial nerve.
- The EPLA gives the most extensive exposure (94%) of the radial shaft.
- When plating the humeral shaft under the radial nerve, surgeons should make a note in their operative reports of the exact location of the nerve (by screw hole number in the plate).

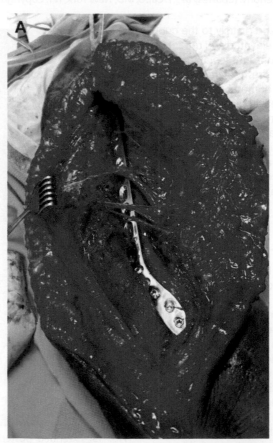

Fig. 14. (*A*) A plate specifically designed for the extended posterior-lateral approach is seen stabilizing a distal humeral shaft fracture. The radial nerve proper and cutaneous nerves lie over the plate. Preoperative (*B*) and postoperative (*C*) radiographs showing a distal third humeral shaft fracture with a butterfly fragment stabilized with a precontoured J plate. The distal aspect has multiple locking screws placed for added stability. (*Courtesy of* J.T. Capo, MD, New York, NY. Copyright © 2014. All Rights Reserved.)

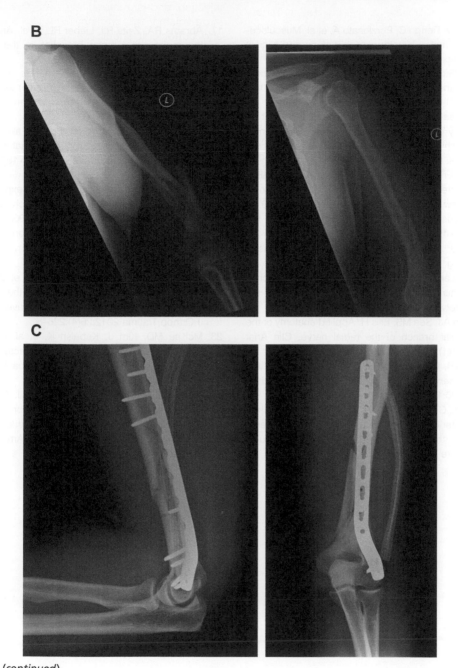

Fig. 14. (*continued*)

REFERENCES

1. Moore KL, Dalley AF, Agur AM, editors. Clinically oriented anatomy 7th edition. Baltimore (MD): Lippincott Williams & Wilkins; 2014.
2. Burkhead WZ Jr, Scheinberg RR, Box G. Surgical anatomy of the axillary nerve. J Shoulder Elbow Surg 1992;1(1):31–6.
3. Uz A, Apaydin N, Bozkurt M, et al. The anatomic branch pattern of the axillary nerve. J Shoulder Elbow Surg 2007;16(2):240–4.
4. Mazurek MT, Shin AY. Upper extremity peripheral nerve anatomy: current concepts and applications. Clin Orthop Relat Res 2001;(383):7–20.
5. Remerand F, Laulan J, Couvret C, et al. Is the musculocutaneous nerve really in the coracobrachialis muscle when performing an axillary block? An ultrasound study. Anesth Analg 2010;110(6):1729–34.
6. Krishnamurthy A, Nayak SR, Venkatraya Prabhu L, et al. The branching pattern and communications of the musculocutaneous nerve. J Hand Surg Eur Vol 2007;32:560–2.

7. Macchi V, Tiengo C, Porzionato A, et al. Musculocutaneous nerve: histotopographic study and clinical
implications. Clin Anat 2007;20:400–6.

8. Guerri-Guttenberg RA, Ingolotti M. Classifying musculocutaneous nerve variations. Clin Anat 2009;
22(6):671–83.

9. Contreras MG, Warner MA, Charboneau WJ, et al.
Anatomy of the ulnar nerve at the elbow: potential
relationship of acute ulnar neuropathy to gender differences. Clin Anat 1998;11:372–8.

10. Gabel GT, Amadio PC. Reoperation for failed
decompression of the ulnar nerve in the region of
the elbow. J Bone Joint Surg Am 1990;72:213–9.

11. De Jesus R, Dellon AL. Historical origin of the
"Arcade of Struthers". J Hand Surg 2003;28:528–31.

12. Terry RJ. A study of the supracondyloid process in
the living. Am J Phys Anthropol 1921;4.

13. Uhl RL, Larosa JM, Sibeni T, et al. Posterior approaches
to the humerus: when should you worry about the
radial nerve? J Orthop Trauma 1996;10:338–40.

14. Robson AJ, See MS, Ellis H. Applied anatomy of the
superficial branch of the radial nerve. Clin Anat
2008;21(1):38–45.

15. Guse TR, Ostrum RF. The surgical anatomy of the
radial nerve around the humerus. Clin Orthop
1995;320:149–53.

16. Low CK, Chew JT, Mitra AK. A surgical approach to
the posterior interosseous branch of the radial nerve
through the brachioradialis: a cadaveric study.
Singapore Med J 1994;35:394–6.

17. Abrams RA, Zeits RJ, Lieber RL, et al. Anatomy of
the radial nerve motor branches in the forearm.
J Hand Surg 1997;22:232–7.

18. Kameda Y. An anomalous muscle (accessory
subscapularis-teres-latissimus muscle) in the axilla
penetrating the brachial plexus in man. Acta Anat
(Basel) 1976;96(4):513–33.

19. Yamaguchi K, Sweet FA, Bindra R, et al. The extra-
osseous and intraosseous arterial anatomy of the
adult elbow. J Bone Joint Surg Am 1997;79(11):
1653–62.

20. Hoppenfeld S, deBoer P. Surgical exposures in
orthopaedics: the anatomic approach. Baltimore
(MD): Lippincott Williams & Wilkins; 2003.

21. Zlotolow DA, Catalano LW 3rd, Barron OA, et al.
Surgical exposures of the humerus. J Am Acad
Orthop Surg 2006;14(13):754–65.

22. Seigerman DA, Choung EW, Yoon RS, et al. Identification of the radial nerve during the posterior
approach to the humerus: a cadaveric study.
J Orthop Trauma 2012;26(4):226–8.

23. McKee MD, Kim J, Kebaish K, et al. Functional
outcome after open supracondylar fractures of the
humerus: the effect of surgical approach. J Bone
Joint Surg Br 2000;82(5):646–51.

24. Gerwin M, Hotchkiss RN, Weiland AJ. Alternative
operative exposures of the posterior aspect of
the humeral diaphysis with reference to the
radial nerve. J Bone Joint Surg Am 1996;78:
1690–5.

Exposures of the Elbow

Terry S. Axelrod, MD, MSc, FRCSC

KEYWORDS

- Anatomy • Elbow • Surgical exposures • Medial • Lateral

KEY POINTS

- Basic anatomy of the elbow is described.
- Surgical exposures to the elbow that are commonly used are lateral, posterior, and medial.
- Advantages and disadvantages of each exposure are described.
- Clinical application of the anatomy and exposures are provided.

The bony anatomy of the elbow is well defined, but complex. The elbow consists of 3 major bones and 3 interrelated joints.

The bone structure allows the simple hinge motion of flexion and extension, but allows for forearm rotation through the radial-capitellar and proximal radioulnar joints (**Fig. 1**).

The bony landmarks are noted in **Fig. 2**.

The 3 joints work in concert in order to allow the degrees of motion of the elbow.[1] The thick vertical ridges of bone, the medial and lateral columns, provide structural support to the joint. They are the structures that cradle the articular segments, the trochlea, and the capitellum (**Figs. 3** and **4**).

Ligamentous structures are the key to the stability and the mobility of the elbow. The medial collateral ligament is a short, stout structure consisting of 3 bundles: the anterior, posterior, and the transverse ligament or bundle. The medial collateral ligament (MCL) forms a triangular structure, originating on the inferior aspect of the medial epicondyle, with the anterior bundle inserting into the anterior aspect of the sublime tubercle of the proximal ulna (**Fig. 5**).

The posterior bundle inserts toward the posterior aspect of the tubercle. These two bundles play different roles in providing stability in flexion and extension of the elbow (**Figs. 6** and **7**).

On the lateral side, the lateral collateral ligament originates on the distal aspect of the lateral epicondyle, inserting in a fanlike fashion into the annular ligament surrounding the radial head (**Fig. 8**), which allows indirect insertion into the proximal radius and, through the insertion of the annular ligament, into the proximal lateral ulna.

THE NEUROLOGIC ANATOMY OF THE ARM AND ELBOW

The 2 major nerves of the arm that course in the regions of the commonly described surgical exposures to the elbow are the radial and the ulnar nerves.

The radial nerve appears in the midposterior arm between the medial and lateral heads of the triceps, coursing distally in the spiral groove of the humerus. It travels from posterior to anterior, piercing through the lateral intermuscular septum approximately 10 cm proximal to the elbow joint, and emerging between the brachialis and brachioradialis muscle groups (**Fig. 9**). This distal location is the easiest location in which to find this nerve.

The ulnar nerve is found in the midarm, initially anterior to the intermuscular septum. It passes into the posterior compartment of the arm approximately 8 cm proximal to the medial epicondyle, then coursing into the cubital tunnel (**Fig. 10**). Once distal to the tunnel, it passes between the 2 heads of origin of the flexor carpi ulnaris (FCU) muscle, giving off the motor branch to the FCU shortly thereafter.

Division of Orthopaedic Surgery, University of Toronto, Sunnybrook Health Sciences Centre, MG301-2075 Bayview Avenue, Toronto, ON M4N 3M5, Canada
E-mail address: terry.axelrod@sunnybrook.ca

Hand Clin 30 (2014) 415–425
http://dx.doi.org/10.1016/j.hcl.2014.08.001
0749-0712/14/$ – see front matter © 2014 Elsevier Inc. All rights reserved.

hand.theclinics.com

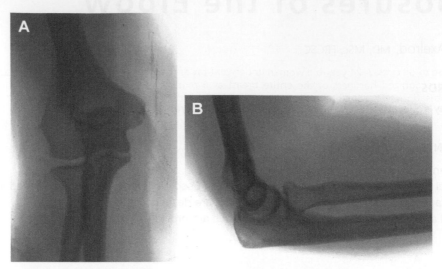

Fig. 1. Anteroposterior (A) and lateral (B) radiograph projections of a normal elbow.

SURGICAL EXPOSURES OF THE ELBOW

The most common posterior exposures to the elbow joint are discussed here, as well as the medial and lateral approaches. The anterior exposure is not reviewed.

POSTERIOR EXPOSURES TO THE ELBOW

The standard posterior exposures to the elbow are the olecranon osteotomy, the triceps-sparing exposure (otherwise known as the triceps-on

exposure), the Mayo (Morrey and colleagues)[2] medial triceps elevation, and the triceps split exposures. The advantages and disadvantages to each are discussed later.

The olecranon osteotomy provides the most extensive exposure to the distal humerus, allowing visualization around and to the front of the joint, which is of particular use with fractures that involve the anterior aspects of the joint surfaces (eg, coronoid shear fractures). The exposure is limited in the ability to extend proximally because of the course of the radial nerve, resulting in a problem if traction is applied to this structure when reflecting the distal triceps too far proximally.

The technique for performing the osteotomy begins with a posterior midline incision. Mobilize the ulnar nerve as per standard techniques distally to the level of the motor branch to the FCU. A longitudinal split in the triceps fascia is created to join the medial distal border of the muscle to the midportion of the olecranon articular surface (**Fig. 11**). The fascial split on the lateral side is similar, carried from the distal lateral muscle ridge of the triceps to the floor of the olecranon. Some fibers of the anconeus muscle are cut with this dissection.

Once the midpoint of the olecranon is established for the osteotomy, place a protective sponge or instrument across the joint surface (see **Fig. 11**). The osteotomy is usually made as a chevron, with the apex distally. The cut is made with a small oscillating saw, completing it with an osteotome. The use of the osteotome reduces the amount of articular cartilage damage at the joint surface, as well as eliminating cartilage loss caused by the kerf of the saw blade.

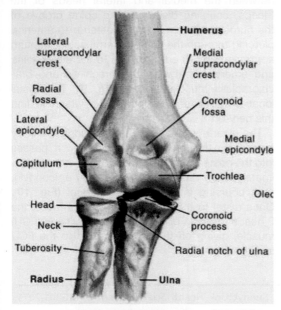

Fig. 2. Anatomic bone structures of the elbow. (*Netter illustration from* www.netterimages.com. © Elsevier Inc. All rights reserved.)

Anatomy

Three Joints

1. **Ulnohumeral**
2. **Radiocapitellar**
3. **Proximal Radioulnar**

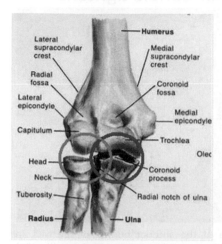

Fig. 3. The 3 principal joints of the elbow. (*Netter illustration from* www.netterimages.com. © Elsevier Inc. All rights reserved.)

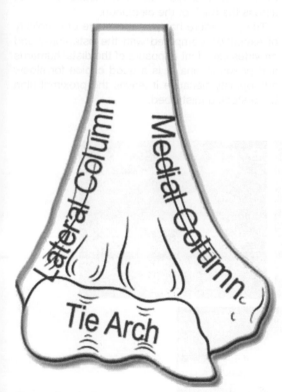

Fig. 4. The thick medial and lateral bone columns support the articular segment. (*From* Singh AP. Fractures of distal third humerus-diagnosis and treatment. BoneandSpine.com project. Available at: http://boneandspine.com/fractures-of-distal-third-humerus-diagnosis-and-treatment/#comment-1649. Accessed July 28, 2014.)

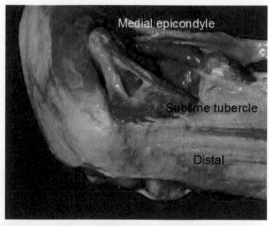

Fig. 5. Medial collateral ligament. (*Courtesy of* A. Gupta, MD, Louisville, KY.)

In flexion: Posterior Bundle tightens

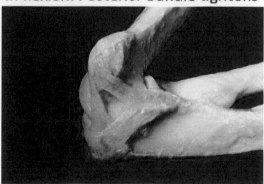

Fig. 6. Role of the posterior bundle of the MCL in flexion. (*Courtesy of* A. Gupta, MD, Louisville, KY.)

Into extension: anterior bundle tightens

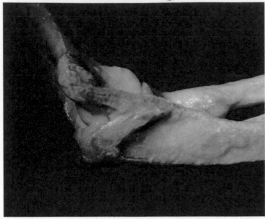

Fig. 7. Role of the anterior bundle of the MCL in extension. (*Courtesy of* A. Gupta, MD, Louisville, KY.)

Once completed, the combined flap of the proximal olecranon and distal triceps is elevated proximally, teasing away the medial and lateral muscle fibers as needed.

Reduction and fixation of the osteotomy at the end of the procedure can be done with standard K wire–based tension band technique, use of a small plate (**Figs. 13** and **14**), or (less favorably) with a large intramedullary screw in combination with a tension band wire around the distal triceps.[3]

The triceps-sparing, or triceps-on, exposure uses the same medial and lateral windows as the olecranon osteotomy; however, the surgeon does not cut the bone (**Fig. 15**). With adequate mobilization of the medial and lateral windows, the distal humerus can be visualized fairly well. The idea is to look across the joint from side to side as needed (**Fig. 16**).

This exposure has one distinct advantage, in that the triceps insertion is not disturbed, reducing the possibility of triceps tendon avulsion, weakness, and so forth.

The disadvantage lies in the limited joint visualization. With this limitation, this exposure, in the author's opinion, is not suitable for dealing with anything other than an extra-articular distal humerus fracture, or perhaps a fracture with a single, simple, minimally displaced split into the joint. It is ideal for primary total elbow arthroplasty for complex fracture management.

The Mayo or Bryan-Morrey[2] exposure to the elbow is based on an elevation of the triceps tendon as a single flap from medial to lateral across the back of the olecranon.

The procedure has the advantage of simplicity of execution compared with the osteotomy and provides excellent exposure of the distal humerus and proximal ulna. It is a good choice for elbow arthroplasty because it leaves the proximal ulna bone stock undisturbed.

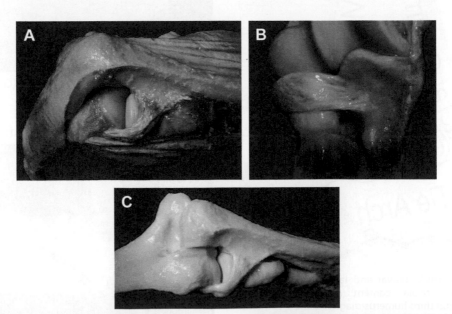

Fig. 8. The origin of the lateral collateral ligament, along with the insertion into the annular ligament of the proximal radius. (*A*) The annular ligament then inserts into the anterior (*B*) and posterior (*C*) aspects of the proximal, lateral ulna. (*Courtesy of* A. Gupta, MD, Louisville, KY.)

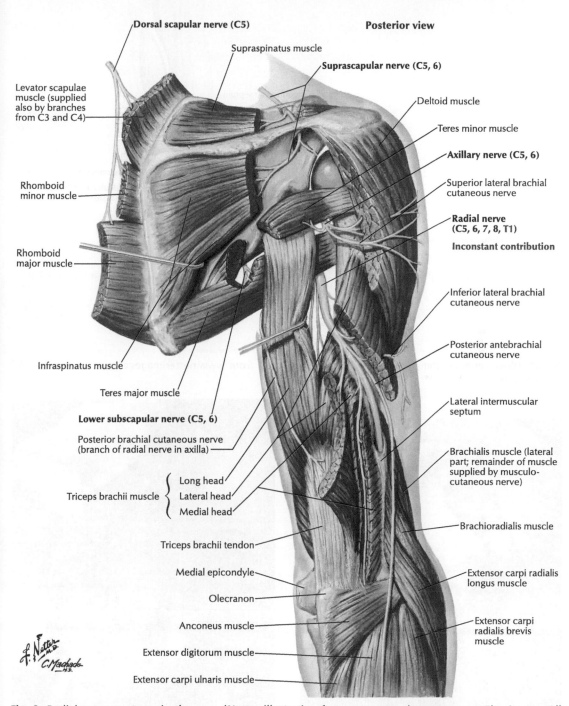

Posterior view

Dorsal scapular nerve (C5)

Supraspinatus muscle

Suprascapular nerve (C5, 6)

Levator scapulae muscle (supplied also by branches from C3 and C4)

Deltoid muscle

Teres minor muscle

Axillary nerve (C5, 6)

Superior lateral brachial cutaneous nerve

Rhomboid minor muscle

Radial nerve (C5, 6, 7, 8, T1)

Inconstant contribution

Rhomboid major muscle

Inferior lateral brachial cutaneous nerve

Posterior antebrachial cutaneous nerve

Infraspinatus muscle

Teres major muscle

Lateral intermuscular septum

Lower subscapular nerve (C5, 6)

Posterior brachial cutaneous nerve (branch of radial nerve in axilla)

Brachialis muscle (lateral part; remainder of muscle supplied by musculo-cutaneous nerve)

Triceps brachii muscle { Long head / Lateral head / Medial head

Brachioradialis muscle

Triceps brachii tendon

Extensor carpi radialis longus muscle

Medial epicondyle

Olecranon

Extensor carpi radialis brevis muscle

Anconeus muscle

Extensor digitorum muscle

Extensor carpi ulnaris muscle

Fig. 9. Radial nerve anatomy in the arm. (*Netter illustration from* www.netterimages.com. © Elsevier Inc. All rights reserved.)

The exposure of the joint can be reasonably good, allowing the surgeon to fix some more challenging intra-articular fractures with this approach.

The difficulty with this choice is that the triceps tendon is extremely thin at the central portion of its insertion into the proximal ulna. There is often a large defect created in the central portion of the tendon with this exposure, making a secure closure more difficult. Morrey suggested that a flap using the fascia of the anconeus can help to

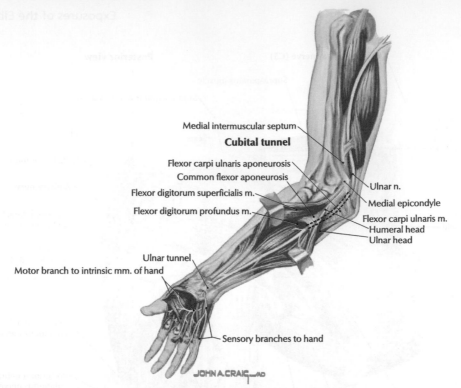

Medial intermuscular septum

Cubital tunnel

Flexor carpi ulnaris aponeurosis

Common flexor aponeurosis

Flexor digitorum superficialis m.

Flexor digitorum profundus m.

Ulnar n.

Medial epicondyle

Flexor carpi ulnaris m.

Humeral head

Ulnar head

Ulnar tunnel

Motor branch to intrinsic mm. of hand

Sensory branches to hand

JOHN A.CRAIG_AD

Fig. 10. Ulnar nerve anatomy in the arm. (*Netter illustration from* www.netterimages.com. © Elsevier Inc. All rights reserved.)

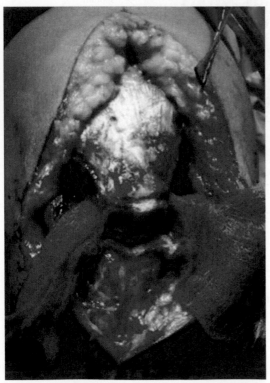

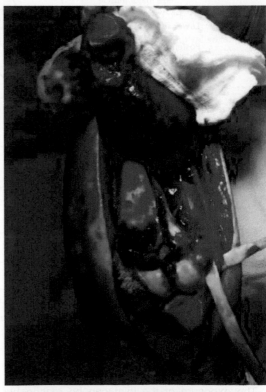

Fig. 11. Technique for performing the olecranon osteotomy. (*Courtesy of* AO Foundation, Davos, Switzerland. AO surgery reference. Available at: https://www2.aofoundation.org/wps/portal/surgery.)

Fig. 12. Exposure following osteotomy with proximal retraction of the triceps flap. Note the excellent view of the joint surface. (*Courtesy of* AO Foundation, Davos, Switzerland. AO surgery reference. Available at: https://www2.aofoundation.org/wps/portal/surgery.)

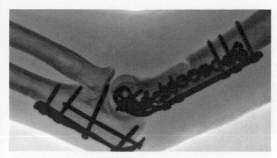

Fig. 13. ORIF of distal humerus fracture seen in **Fig. 12,** closure of olecranon osteotomy using a plate and screws. (*Courtesy of* AO Foundation, Davos, Switzerland. AO surgery reference. Available at: https://www2.aofoundation.org/wps/portal/surgery.)

reinforce this repair. This approach to the elbow may be associated with more failures of the triceps repair.

The triceps split is an extensive exposure that can be used to visualize the back of the arm from just below the deltoid insertion to the distal aspect of the ulna. The split uses long flaps of the triceps tendon insertion and aponeurosis to allow the surgeon to reflect the triceps mass anteriorly, exposing the distal humerus extremely well.

The fascial closure is very secure to bone, reducing the chance of a failure of the triceps repair at the completion of the procedure.

This exposure is done by mobilizing the ulnar nerve as described earlier. The midline of the triceps insertion into the olecranon is identified and serves as the guide for the longitudinal cut into the tendon. The tendon is sharply split proximally,

being aware of the radial nerve location when approaching the midarm level.

The key to success with the distal triceps split is to continue the sharp dissection along the subcutaneous border of the ulna to at least 8 to 10 cm distal to the tip of the olecranon. The elevation of the triceps tendon is done with sharp scalpel dissection because use of cautery vaporizes the tendon material, leaving a defect at the time of repair.

At repair, drill holes are made in the ulna allowing for suture repair of the tendon back to bone. Side-to-side advancement of the medial and lateral flaps serves to reinforce the tendon bulk.

This exposure provides an excellent view of the distal humerus, including the joint. It is better for a more complex intra-articular distal humerus fracture than the triceps-on exposure. It is a little more limited for viewing the joint surface and, in particular, the anterior aspect of the joint. The view is not as good as with an olecranon osteotomy.

The exposure can be extended proximally, which is ideal for fractures that extend more proximally up the humerus or combination fractures of the diaphyseal humerus plus supracondylar. It can be used very well for total elbow arthroplasty.

MEDIAL EXPOSURES OF THE ELBOW

Medial exposures to the elbow are typically indicated for management of medial collateral ligament injuries that require repair, as can be associated with the so-called terrible triad elbow bone and soft tissue fracture dislocation. In addition, this exposure can be used for approaching the medial coronoid facet fracture that requires

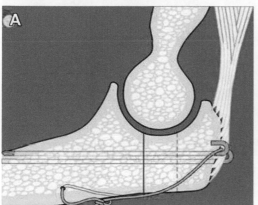
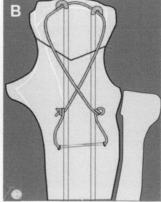

Fig. 14. (*A, B*) Repair of the olecranon osteotomy with the tension band wire technique. (*Courtesy of* AO Foundation, Davos, Switzerland. AO surgery reference. Available at: https://www2.aofoundation.org/wps/portal/surgery.)

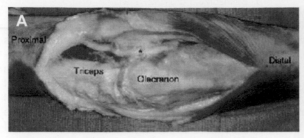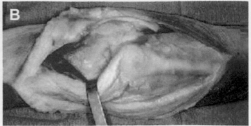

Fig. 15. (*A*, *B*) Triceps-on exposure. (*From* Cheung EV, Steinmann SP. Surgical approaches to the elbow. J Am Acad Orthop Surg 2009;17:325–33; with permission.)

reduction and fixation. Cheung and Steinmann[4] provide an excellent description of the medial surgical exposures to the elbow.

The exposure is limited, not being extensile distally.

The approach can be performed by either a long posterior elbow skin incision, elevating a medial flap, or surgeons can use a medial incision halfway between the medial epicondyle and the olecranon.

It is very important that the ulnar nerve is identified and mobilized generously proximally and distally.

The FCU fascia is split during the ulnar nerve mobilization. The interval between the 2 heads of the FCU is developed, taking the humeral origin off the proximal ulna as a full-thickness flap. This step brings the surgeon down to the anterior half of the proximal ulna and thus the coronoid process. The exposure is kept anterior to the sublime tubercle and, thus, the medial collateral ligament (**Fig. 17**).

In situations of MCL injury the exposure is usually created by the injury, once the ulnar nerve is mobilized (**Fig. 18**).

Dr Robert Hotchkiss[4,5] described a variant of this medial elbow exposure in which the approach is not between the heads of the FCU, but rather over the top of the humeral origin portion of the common flexor pronator muscle mass. This variant requires the surgeon to resect the distal portion of the medial intermuscular septum and then elevate the common flexor pronator muscle origin off the medial distal humerus, leaving most of the humeral origin of the FCU still attached to the bone. This exposure provides a good view of the anterior capsule and the coronoid process, although less so of the sublime tubercle and the MCL. Anatomic

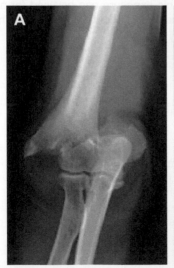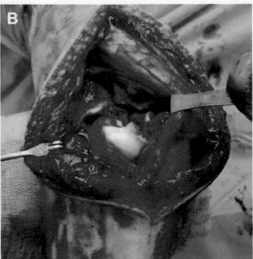

Fig. 16. (*A*, *B*) Clinical case of extra-articular distal humerus fracture exposed using the triceps-on technique. Visualization is achieved by elevating the triceps and looking across the joint from side to side. (*Courtesy of* AO Foundation, Davos, Switzerland. AO surgery reference. Available at: https://www2.aofoundation.org/wps/portal/surgery.)

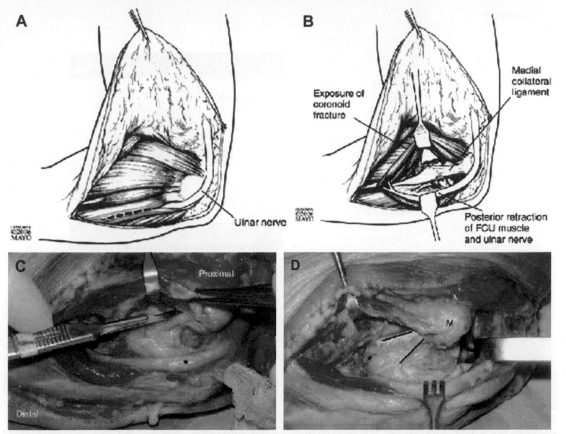

Fig. 17. (*A–D*) Exposure of the medial collateral ligament of the elbow, using the split FCU technique. C * Ulnar nerve, D * medial collateral ligament. (*Courtesy of* Mayo Foundation for Medical Education and Research; with permission; all rights reserved; and *From* Cheung EV, Steinmann SP. Surgical approaches to the elbow. J Am Acad Orthop Surg 2009;17:325–33; with permission.)

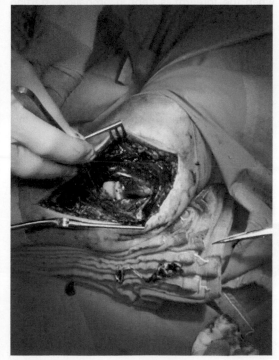

Fig. 18. A 19-year-old man had an acute varus injury to his elbow resulting in a complete avulsion of his MCL off of the distal humerus. The medial exposure is shown.

studies by Huh and colleagues[6] suggest that this exposure provides a more restricted view than the traditional FCU split approach.

LATERAL EXPOSURES OF THE ELBOW

The 2 exposures most frequently used for approaching the lateral side of the elbow are the Kaplan[7] (**Fig. 19**) and Kocher (**Fig. 20**) exposures. Both are used for exposing lateral column fractures of the distal humerus, capitellar fractures, and most commonly for access to the proximal radius. Through these exposures, the surgeon can access radial head and/or neck fractures for fixation or arthroplasty. Either can be used to address lateral collateral ligament injuries, either in isolation or in combination with radial head disorders.

Both exposures use lateral skin incisions, beginning just proximal to the lateral epicondyle and curving distally to a region approximately halfway between the radial head and the olecranon. With the Kaplan[7] exposure the incision tends to be a little more anterior at the distal portion.

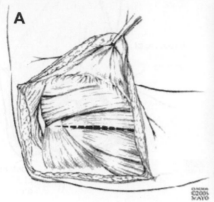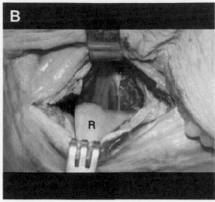

Fig. 19. (*A, B*) Kaplan[7] exposure. (*Courtesy of* Mayo Foundation for Medical Education and Research; with permission; all rights reserved; and *From* Cheung EV, Steinmann SP. Surgical approaches to the elbow. J Am Acad Orthop Surg 2009;17:325–33; with permission.)

The Kaplan[7] exposure (see **Fig. 19**) is a more direct approach to the lateral elbow, developing the interval between the extensor carpi radialis brevis and the extensor digitorum communis tendons. This thick, almost pure tendon strip is found between the muscle belly origins. It is directly over the radial head distally.

The Kaplan[7] exposure is simple, but it is a little more limiting in that the surgeon splits into the supinator muscle going distally beyond the radial neck. This split can place the posterior interosseous nerve (PIN) at risk for injury. When using this exposure, it is prudent to tease apart the proximal portion of the supinator to identify the fibers of the PIN in order to protect them. Keeping the forearm in pronation during the exposure may also limit the risk of harm to the nerve.

The Kocher exposure was first described in 1911 by T. Kocher[8] in his textbook of operative surgery. This exposure uses a similar skin incision to that of the Kaplan[7] exposure, perhaps keeping the distal extent of the incision a little more posterior.

The exposure develops the interval between the anconeus muscle and the extensor carpi ulnaris muscle (see **Fig. 20**). During the deep part of this dissection, the surgeon can elevate the supinator muscle off the proximal radius when the forearm is kept in pronation, starting with the deep portion of the supinator, near the proximal ulna, which allows reasonable exposure of the proximal radius, elevating off the supinator and, with it, the PIN distal to the radial neck. According to Mekhail and colleagues,[9] surgeons can safely extend the approach a few centimeters (up to 6 cm of the proximal radius exposed) with the Kocher exposure following this technique.

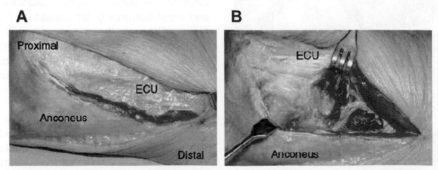

Fig. 20. (*A, B*) Kocher exposure. ECU, extensor carpi ulnaris. (*From* Cheung EV, Steinmann SP. Surgical approaches to the elbow. J Am Acad Orthop Surg 2009;17:325–33; with permission.)

REFERENCES

1. AO Foundation AO surgery reference. Available at: https://www2.aofoundation.org/wps/portal/surgery. Accessed July 13, 2014.
2. Bryan RS, Morrey BF. Extensive posterior exposure of the elbow: a triceps sparing approach. Clin Orthop 1982;166:188.
3. AO Trauma North America lecture archives. Available at: https://www.aona.org. Accessed July 13, 2014.
4. Cheung EV, Steinmann SP. Surgical approaches to the elbow. J Am Acad Orthop Surg 2009;17:325–33.
5. Kasparyan NG, Hotchkiss RN. Dynamic skeletal fixation in the upper extremity. Hand Clin 1997;13(4): 643–63.
6. Huh J, Krueger CA, Medvecky MJ, et al, Skeletal Trauma Research Consortium. Medial elbow exposure for coronoid fractures: FCU-split versus over-the-top. J Orthop Trauma 2013;27(12):730–4.
7. Kaplan EB. Surgical approach to the proximal end of the radius and its use in fractures of the head and neck of the radius. J Bone Joint Surg 1941; 23:86–92.
8. Kocher T. Textbook of operative surgery. 3rd edition. New York: Macmillan; 1911. p. 314–8.
9. Mekhail AO, Ebraheim NA, Jackson WT, et al. Vulnerability of the posterior interosseous nerve during proximal radius exposures. Clin Orthop 1995;315:199–208.

Exposure of the Forearm and Distal Radius

Melissa A. Klausmeyer, MD[a], Chaitanya Mudgal, MD[b],*

KEYWORDS

- Henry approach • Thompson approach • Flexor carpi radialis approach
- Dorsal distal radius approach • Distal radius approach

KEY POINTS

- The use of internervous planes allow access to the underlying bone without risk of denervating the overlying muscles.
- The choice of approach is based on the injury pattern and need for exposure.
- The Henry and Thompson approaches are useful for radial shaft fractures.
- The distal radius can be approached volarly through the flexor carpi radialis (FCR) approach or dorsally through the extended Thompson approach.
- The extended FCR approach is useful for intraarticular fractures of the distal radius as well as malunions and subacute fractures.

INTRODUCTION

Safe operative approaches to the bones of the forearm and wrist include the use of internervous planes. These planes lie between muscles that are innervated by different nerves. By utilizing these planes for dissection, extensive mobilization of muscles and therefore large areas of exposure may be obtained without the risk of muscle denervation.

A successful operative plan also must include consideration of the soft tissues, particularly flexion creases. Elective incisions should not cross the wrist crease or antecubital fossa perpendicularly. Scars contract with time, and incisions that cross these creases can result in loss of extension secondary to scar contracture on the flexion surface. If crossing the flexion crease is necessary, a transverse or zig-zag incision should be incorporated to prevent this scar contracture.

ANATOMY OF THE FOREARM
Muscles

The muscles of the forearm are split into 4 compartments: The superficial volar, the deep volar, the extensor, and the mobile wad (**Table 1**). The median nerve supplies all of the volar muscles of the forearm except the ulnar half of the flexor digitorum profundus and the flexor carpi ulnaris that are supplied by the ulnar nerve. The radial nerve proper supplies the brachioradialis and extensor carpi radialis longus. The posterior interosseous branch of the radial nerve supplies the other muscles of the dorsal compartment. Variations do exist, notably the innervation of the extensor carpi radialis brevis (ECRB), which is supplied by the superficial (sensory) branch of the radial nerve in 58% of cases.[1]

Arteries

The brachial artery is the main arterial supply to the forearm and distal structures. Below the elbow

The authors have nothing to disclose.
[a] Division of Plastic and Reconstructive Surgery, Department of Orthopedic Surgery, University of Colorado Hospital, Mail Stop C309, 12631 East 17th Avenue, Aurora, CO 80045, USA; [b] Hand and Upper Extremity Service, Department of Orthopedics, Harvard Medical School, Yawkey 2C, 55 Fruit Street, Boston, MA 02114, USA
* Corresponding author.
E-mail address: cmudgal@partners.org

Hand Clin 30 (2014) 427–433
http://dx.doi.org/10.1016/j.hcl.2014.07.002

Table 1
Four compartments of the forearm

	Origin	Insertion	Innervation
Superficial volar forearm			
Pronator teres	Medial epicondyle	Mid third of radius	Median
Flexor carpi radialis	Medial epicondyle	Base of second MC	Median
Palmaris longus	Medial epicondyle	Palmar fascia of hand	Median
Flexor carpi ulnaris	Medial epicondyle	Pisiform/base of fifth MC	Ulnar
Flexor digitorum superficialis	Medial epicondyle	Base of middle phalanx of index, long, ring, small	Median
Deep volar forearm			
Flexor digitorum profundus	Ulna/interosseus membrane	Base of distal phalanx of index, long, ring, small	Median (anterior interosseous branch) (index, long)/ulnar nerve (ring, small)
Flexor pollicis longus	Distal third of radius	Base of thumb distal phalanx	Median (anterior interosseous branch)
Pronator quadratus	Distal third of ulna	Distal third of radius	Median (anterior interosseous branch)
Dorsal forearm			
Abductor pollicis longus	Mid-third dorsal radius	Radial base of thumb MC	Radial (posterior interosseous branch)
Extensor pollicis brevis	Mid-third dorsal radius	Dorsal base of thumb proximal phalanx	Radial (posterior interosseous branch)
Extensor pollicis longus	Dorsal ulna	Dorsal base of thumb distal phalanx	Radial (posterior interosseous branch)
Extensor digitorum communis	Lateral epicondyle	Dorsal base of distal phalanx of index, long, ring, small	Radial (posterior interosseous branch)
Extensor indicis proprius	Dorsal ulna	Dorsal base of index distal phalanx	Radial (posterior interosseous branch)
Extensor digiti quinti	Lateral epicondyle	Dorsal base of small distal phalanx	Radial (posterior interosseous branch)
Extensor carpi ulnaris	Lateral epicondyle	Dorsal base of small MC	Radial (posterior interosseous branch)
Supinator	Lateral epicondyle	Proximal third of radius	Radial (posterior interosseous branch)
Mobile wad			
Brachioradialis	Lateral condyle humerus	Distal radius styloid	Radial
Extensor carpi radialis longus	Lateral condyle humerus	Dorsal base of second MC	Radial
Extensor carpi radialis brevis	Lateral condyle humerus	Dorsal base of 3rd MC	Radial (posterior interosseous branch)

Abbreviation: MC, metacarpal.

crease and distal to the biceps aponeurosis, it divides into the radial and ulnar branches. The radial artery travels between the brachioradialis and pronator teres proximally and becomes more superficial distally, where it lies between the brachioradialis and flexor carpi radialis (FCR). The ulnar artery lies superficial to the flexor digitorum profundus and between the flexor carpi ulnaris ulnarly and the flexor digitorum superficialis radially.

Nerves

Three main nerves supply the forearm: The radial, median, and ulnar. The median nerve enters the forearm between the 2 heads of the pronator teres. It travels deep to the flexor digitorum superficialis. Distally, it becomes more superficial and may be mistaken for the palmaris longus with potentially devastating consequences. The radial nerve branches into the superficial sensory and deep motor branches (posterior interosseus nerve [PIN]) just proximal to the ECRB at the level of the lateral epicondyle. The sensory branch exits from under the brachioradialis at the middle of the forearm, about 8 to 10 cm proximal to the radial styloid.[2] The deep branch enters the supinator as it courses from the anterior to the posterior surface of the forearm. The ulnar nerve enters the forearm between the 2 heads of the flexor carpi ulnaris. It travels between the flexor digitorum superficialis and the flexor carpi ulnaris as it courses distally. The dorsal branch of the ulnar nerve arises about 8 cm proximal to the pisiform

and crosses the subcutaneous border of the ulna. It crosses dorsally about 5 cm proximal to the pisiform.[3]

HENRY APPROACH

This approach utilizes the internervous plane between the brachioradialis (radial nerve) and pronator teres (median nerve) proximally, or the brachioradialis (radial nerve) and FCR (median nerve) distally. It is utilized primarily for fractures of the radius, particularly the distal half (**Fig. 1**), as well as for radial sensory nerve decompression (Wartenberg syndrome) and to approach the bicipital tuberosity of the radius from the volar aspect.

The forearm is placed in the supinated position. The incision is made just proximal to the wrist flexion crease and radial to the FCR (see **Fig. 1**E). The incision extends proximally, parallel to this tendon. The incision ends distal to the elbow flexion crease and just lateral to the biceps tendon. After dividing the fascia, the interval between the brachioradialis and the FCR is

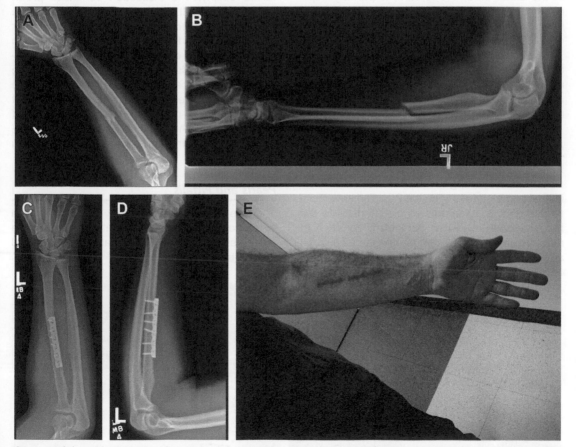

Fig. 1. PA (*A*) and lateral (*B*) radiographs demonstrating displaced midshaft radius fracture. PA (*C*) and lateral (*D*) radiographs of case 1 after plate fixation via a Henry approach. Note the volar placement of the plate. (*E*) Surgical scar of Henry approach used in case 1.

developed distally. Care is taken to not drift ulnarly to the FCR to avoid inadvertent damage to the median nerve. The superficial radial sensory nerve exits from under the brachioradialis at the mid forearm level, approximately 8 to 10 cm proximal to the radial styloid. Proximally, the dissection continues between the pronator teres and the brachioradialis. The braches of the radial artery to the brachioradialis may be ligated to improve retraction of the brachioradialis in the radial direction. The dissection continues deep by following the bicep tendon on the bicipital tuberosity. The bursa is incised radial to the tendon to avoid the radial artery, which runs ulnarly. The elbow is flexed to allow for improved retraction of the brachioradialis. The forearm is supinated to displace the posterior interosseous nerve radially and to visualize the insertion of the supinator. The supinator is incised, and elevated subperiosteally.

In the middle third, the forearm is pronated to visualize the insertion of the pronator teres, which can be elevated to achieve access to the radius. In the distal third, the forearm is partially supinated and the dissection continues along the lateral aspect of the radius, lateral to the pronator quadratus.[4]

Disadvantages of this approach include the need for stripping of soft tissues, which can delay return of hand function. Also, a volarly placed plate on the proximal third of the radius may block pronation of the forearm.

Pearls and Pitfalls

Drifting ulnarly to the FCR can damage the median nerve. Not dissecting the supinator in the subperiosteal plane can damage the PIN. The superficial radial nerve is vulnerable as it runs deep to the brachioradialis, and it is particularly sensitive to retraction and manipulation. Damage to the radial artery as it runs deep to the brachioradialis is another pitfall, because it may not be immediately apparent under tourniquet control.

THOMPSON APPROACH

The Thompson approach utilizes the interneural interval between the ECRB (radial nerve) and the extensor digitorum comminis (EDC; PIN) proximally or the ECRB (radial nerve) and extensor pollicis longus (PIN) distally. This approach is utilized primarily for fractures of the proximal and middle thirds of the distal radius (**Fig. 2**).

The patient's forearm is placed in pronation, and the incision is made along the medial border of the mobile wad of 3 toward the lateral epicondyle proximally and Lister's tubercle distally. Distally, the EDC is identified and the overlying fascia is split on its radial border between the EDC and ECRB in the mobile wad. This interval may be more apparent distally where the APL and EPB cross the radius as opposed to more proximally. The APL and EPB are released along their radial border to avoid denervation, and raised ulnarly. The dissection continues proximally between the ECRB and the EDC. The EDC is then reflected ulnarly, and the supinator is exposed. The PIN must be protected. It can be identified as it exits the 2 heads of the supinator. The PIN is dissected proximally through the muscle substance of the superficial head. The forearm is pronated to expose the anterior aspect of the radius and move the PIN from the origin of the supinator. The supinator may then be detached by releasing its radial border and raising it ulnarly.[5]

Pearls and Pitfalls

There is a potential for injury of the PIN with dissection through the supinator. Dorsal plate placement may irritate the first and second dorsal compartment tendons.

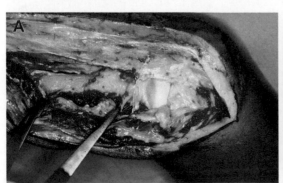
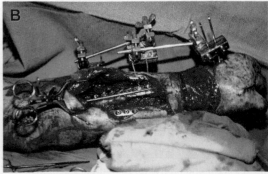

Fig. 2. The Thompson approach is utilized for the exposure of the proximal radius (*A*) and dorsal plate fixation (*B*).

VOLAR APPROACH TO THE DISTAL RADIUS

The distal radius may be approached by the trans-FCR approach. The incision is made directly over the FCR, proximal to the wrist crease (**Fig. 3**A–E). The FCR sheath is opened sharply in line with the tendon on the radial aspect of the sheath to avoid injury to the palmar cutaneous branch of the median nerve (see **Fig. 3**F). This nerve runs along side the FCR tendon and branches from the median nerve approximately 5 cm proximal to the distal wrist crease. The distal

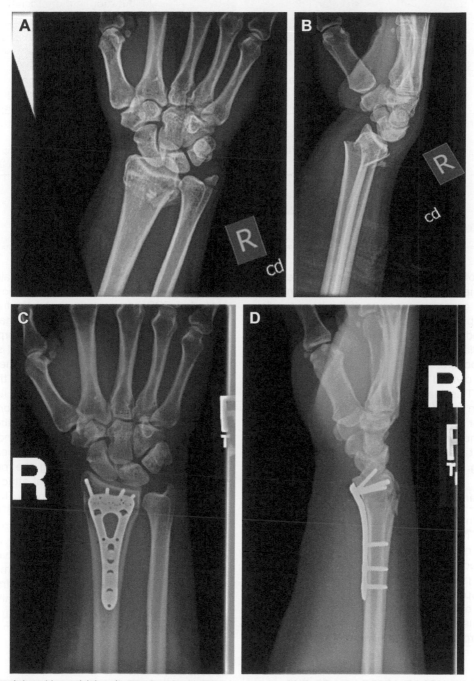

Fig. 3. PA (*A*) and lateral (*B*) radiographs of a displaced intraarticular distal radius fracture. PA (*C*) and lateral (*D*) radiographs demonstrating the volar plate fixation. The extended flexor carpi radialis (FCR) approach is demonstrated. (*E*) Skin incision with FCR tendon sheath exposed. (*F*) The sheath is incised and the tendon retracted radially. (*G*) The pronator quadratus has been elevated, exposing the radius. A hypodermic needle demonstrates the articular space. (*H*) A retractor grasps the radial diaphysis to retract it radially and expose the distal fragments.

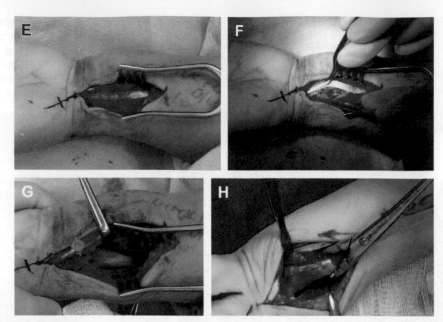

Fig. 3. (*continued*)

aspect of the sheath release extends to the tubercle of the scaphoid. Proximally, it is extended to provide generous exposure of the bone to allow for proper fixation. The FCR tendon is then retracted ulnarly to protect the median nerve. The radial artery is found on the radial aspect of the exposure. The floor of the sheath is then sharply divided and the digit flexors are swept ulnarly.[6] This leads directly into the deep layer between the finger flexors and the pronator quadratus, or Parona's space.[7] The pronator quadratus is then incised in an "L" fashion on its radial and distal aspects and elevated subperiosteally (see **Fig. 3**G).

Pearls and Pitfalls

Damaging the palmar cutaneous branch of the median nerve if the dissection drifts ulnar to the FCR. The radial artery may be inadvertently damaged at the radial aspect of the surgical wound, particularly with sharp retraction. Dissecting subperiosteally too distally along the volar aspect of the radius can potentially disrupt the volar wrist ligaments. Repair of the pronator quadratus protects the volar tendons from the volar hardware.

EXTENDED VOLAR APPROACH TO THE DISTAL RADIUS

The volar approach to the distal radius is useful for fresh fractures (<10 days old) and without severe intraarticular displacement. It does not allow for direct visualization of the joint surface. The extended FCR approach is useful for fractures with organizing hematoma and intraarticular displacement. A zig-zag incision is incorporated across the wrist crease. Then the radial septum is released. Proximally, it separates the flexor and extensor compartments. Distally, the first extensor compartment is released from its deep surface above the insertion of the brachioradialis. The brachioradialis is then released from the radial styloid, allowing for further exposure and eliminating a deforming force. The dissection continues subperiostally and dorsally along the proximal radial fragment, whereas periosteal attachments to the distal fragment(s) are preserved. The proximal fragment is then pronated into the field to allow for visualization of the distal fragments from within the fracture site (see **Fig. 3**H).[8] If necessary, the dorsal periosteum is divided to allow for reduction of the distal fragments.[8,9] Once these are reduced, the proximal fragment is then reduced back into place to allow for fixation. Once complete, the pronator quadratus is repaired over the fixation to protect the flexor tendons.

Pitfalls

Stripping the dorsal periosteum from distal fragments can devitalize the bone. Incomplete release of the brachioradialis and first dorsal compartment can limit reduction.

DORSAL APPROACH TO THE DISTAL RADIUS

This distal radius may be approached dorsally, as an extension of the Thompson approach. A longitudinal incision is made centered over Lister's tubercle. Full-thickness radial and ulnar flaps are developed by elevating the soft tissues off the extensor retinaculum while protecting the superficial branches of the radial and ulnar nerves. The third dorsal compartment is identified and divided longitudinally, and the extensor pollicis longus is released and retracted radially. A partial neurectomy may be performed by dividing the PIN, which is located at the base of the fourth dorsal compartment. The dissection then continues in a subperiosteal fashion both radially under the second and first dorsal compartments and ulnarly under the fourth dorsal compartment. A subperiosteal release of the first dorsal compartment and brachioradialis is also performed from the dorsal approach if necessary to address and reduce radial styloid fracture fragments. If the fracture is intraarticular, a capsular incision is made in an inverted T fashion longitudinally centered over the lunate and transversely along the distal aspect of the lunate. The flaps are elevated and the wrist distracted to inspect the articular surface and for ligamentous injury.[10]

Pitfalls

The sensory branches are at risk if the flaps are not made full thickness when approaching the extensor retinaculum. The terminal branch of the PIN ends at the level of the wrist dorsally in line with the fourth metacarpal. It is easily accessed for partial denervation.

CASES

1. Henry: A 43-year-old man fell from a ladder at work and sustained a displaced midshaft radius fracture. A Henry approach was used for exposure and fixation (see **Fig. 1**).
2. Thompson approach: A 28-year-old man sustained trauma to the forearm after a motorcycle crash, including a proximal radius fracture. The Thompson approach was utilized for proximal radius exposure (see **Fig. 2**).
3. FCR: A 41-year-old woman fell on her outstretched hand while rollerblading. She sustained a dorsally displaced distal radius fracture. An FCR approach was used to apply a volar plate.

REFERENCES

1. Spinner M. Injuries to the major branches of the peripheral nerves of the forearm. Philadelphia: WB Saunders Co; 1972.
2. Abrams RA, Brown RA, Botte MJ. The superficial branch of the radial nerve: an anatomic study with surgical implications. J Hand Surg 1992;17: 1037–41.
3. Botte MJ, Cohen MS, Lavernia CJ, et al. The dorsal branch of the ulnar nerve: an anatomic study. J Hand Surg 1990;15:603–7.
4. Henry AK. Extensile exposure. 2nd edition. Edinburgh (United Kingdom): E&S Livingstone; 1966.
5. Thompson JE. Anatomical methods of approach in operations on the long bones of the extremities. Ann Surg 1918;68:309–29.
6. Jupiter JB, Fernandez DL, Toh CL, et al. Operative treatment of volar intraarticular fractures of the distal end of the radius. J Bone Joint Surg Am 1996;78: 1817–28.
7. Parona F. Dell'oncotomia negli accessi profundi diffuse dell'avambrachio. Milano (Italy): Annali Universali di Medicina e Chirurgia; 1876.
8. Orbay JL, Badia A, Indriago IR, et al. The extended flexor carpi radialis approach: a new perspective for the distal radius fracture. Tech Hand Up Extrem Surg 2001;5:201–11.
9. Wijffels MM, Orbay JL, Indriago I, et al. The extended flexor carpi radialis approach for partially healed malaligned fractures of the distal radius. Injury 2012;43:1204–8.
10. Day CS, Frank OI. Low-profile dorsal plating for dorsally angulated distal radius fractures. Tech Hand Up Extrem Surg 2007;11:142–8.

Exposures of the Wrist and Distal Radioulnar Joint

Kyle D. Bickel, MD

KEYWORDS

- Wrist • DRUJ • Surgical exposure • Technique • Trauma reconstruction

KEY POINTS

- The wrist consists of the 8 carpal bones and their articulations with the distal surfaces of the radius and ulna, as well as the proximal articular surfaces of the metacarpals.
- The distal radioulnar joint (DRUJ) contributes to the stability and function of the wrist.
- The 3 major nerves to the hand—the median, ulnar, and radial nerves—traverse the wrist as they enter the hand. Key anatomic landmarks identify their positions for protection during exposure.
- Standard and alternative exposures of the wrist joint and DRUJ are discussed, with case examples illustrating their use.

ANATOMY OF THE WRIST AND DISTAL RADIOULNAR JOINT

The wrist consists of the 8 carpal bones and their articulations with the distal surfaces of the radius and ulna, as well as the proximal articular surfaces of the metacarpals. The distal radioulnar joint (DRUJ) contributes to the stability and function of the wrist, as well, with stabilization of the ulnar carpus via the triangular fibrocartilage complex (TFCC) and creation of a rotational moment for pronation and supination of the forearm at the DRUJ. The wrist and DRUJ form a highly complex structure, maintained by intrinsic interosseous ligaments between each of the carpal bones, extrinsic radiocarpal and ulnocarpal ligaments, intracapsular ligaments, and the TFCC. The median, ulnar, and radial nerves traverse the wrist and must be protected during surgical exposures. The flexor and extensor tendons to the digits and the wrist surround the joints and also need to be managed carefully to prevent injury during exposures and maintain mobility during healing after surgery. An understanding of these relationships is essential to safe and effective surgical access for the treatment of carpal pathology, ligament injuries, and fracture care.

Skeletal Anatomy

Distal radius and ulna

The distal articular surfaces of the radius and ulna form the pedestal of support for the carpus and the distal locus of rotation during pronation and supination of the forearm. The radius has a series of concavities in its distal articular surface, known as fossae, for support of the scaphoid and lunate. The rim of the radius serves as the site of origin of the extrinsic radiocarpal and radioulnar ligaments (TFCC). The ulnar margin of the radius is concave, with a variable-radius curvature that forms the sigmoid notch for articulation with the distal head of the ulna. This articulation forms the skeletal basis for the DRUJ. The DRUJ is stabilized by the concavity of the sigmoid notch, the dorsal and volar radioulnar ligaments forming the TFCC, the joint capsule, and the distal aspect of the interosseous membrane (**Fig. 1**).

Carpal bones

There are 8 carpal bones, the scaphoid, lunate, triquetrum, pisiform, hamate, capitate, trapezoid, and trapezium. The pisiform is the only carpal bone that does not contribute to articular motion

The author has nothing to disclose.
The Hand Center of San Francisco, 1700 California Street, Suite 450, San Francisco, CA 94109, USA
E-mail address: kbickel@sfhand.com

Hand Clin 30 (2014) 435–444
http://dx.doi.org/10.1016/j.hcl.2014.07.003
0749-0712/14/$ – see front matter

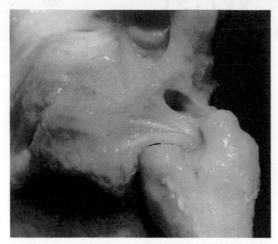

Fig. 1. Cadaveric dissection of the DRUJ stabilizers, the dorsal and volar limbs of the TFCC inserting at the ulnar fovea, and the dorsal capsular attachment of the TFCC. (*Courtesy of* A. Gupta, MD, Louisville, KY.)

of the wrist. It lies palmar to the triquetrum and forms a distal pulley beneath the flexor carpi ulnaris tendon. Each of the 7 articulating carpal bones is connected by a series of intrinsic interosseous ligaments. The bones are contained in 2 rows, a proximal and a distal row. The proximal row (scaphoid, lunate, and triquetrum) articulates with the radius, and indirectly with the distal ulna through the gliding surface of the TFCC central disc. The distal row (hamate, capitate, trapezoid, and trapezium) articulates with the proximal cartilaginous surfaces of the metacarpals. The proximal and distal rows articulate with one another via very complex articular surfaces that contribute significantly to motion of the wrist in both the flexion–extension and the radial–ulnar arcs.

Ligamentous Anatomy

Intrinsic ligaments

Each of the carpal bones has an intrinsic ligamentous connection to the adjacent carpal bones via intrinsic ligaments. The crucial intrinsic ligaments with respect to support and stability are the scapholunate (SLIL) and lunotriquetral interosseous ligaments. The scapholunate (SL) ligament is divided into dorsal, membranous (proximal), and volar segments. The dorsal segment is the primary stabilizer of the SL joint during motion and loading. Disruption of the SLIL may lead to rotational instability of the SL joint, midcarpal joint adaptive instability (dorsal intercalary segment instability), and secondary arthrosis of the radiocarpal and intercarpal joints, (SL advanced collapse). Surgical repair or reconstruction of injuries to the dorsal SLIL is the primary focus of exposure used in treating SL dissociation.

The lunotriquetral interosseous ligament is a shorter and less robust ligament than the SLIL. It

has less distinct dorsal, proximal, and volar segments. Treatment of lunotriquetral interosseous ligaments injuries can be direct, via dorsal wrist exposures, or indirect, via the ulnocarpal ligaments affected by altering radioulnar variance.

Extrinsic ligaments

The extrinsic radiocarpal and ulnocarpal ligaments play an important role in maintaining carpal alignment and stability during wrist motion. The volar radiocarpal ligaments—the radioscaphoid, radioscaphocapitate, long radiolunate, and short radiolunate ligaments—and the volar ulnocarpal ligaments—the ulnocapitate, ulnolunate, and ulnotriquetral ligaments—form a strong, V-shaped sling that maintains radiocarpal alignment during motion and loading of the wrist (**Fig. 2**). These ligaments originate on the volar rim of the radius and ulna, an important end-terminus to any volar exposure of the wrist that must be maintained if radiocarpal stability is to be preserved. The radioscaphoid and radioscaphocapitate ligaments provide a radial tether to the carpus, preventing ulnar shift during weight-bearing and load. They originate from the volar surface of the styloid of the radius and insert on the distal scaphoid and capitate, respectively. The radioscaphocapitate ligament, in particular, acts as a fulcrum for the palmar-dorsal rotation of the scaphoid that occurs with radial and ulnar deviation. This can be a strong deforming force, contributing to flexion

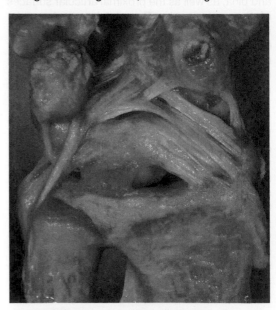

Fig. 2. Cadaveric dissection illustrating the volar extrinsic ligaments of the wrist. The inverted V configuration of the radiocarpal and ulnocarpal ligaments as shown provides a strong ligamentous sling for the carpus, preventing dorsovolar subluxation. (*Courtesy of* A. Gupta, MD, Louisville, KY.)

deformity—the so-called humpback collapse—of the scaphoid in fractures and nonunions.

The dorsal extrinsic ligaments are identifiable organizations of collagen bundles found within the dorsal capsule and attaching to the carpal bones. The major elements are the dorsal radiotriquetral (radiocarpal) ligament and the dorsal intercarpal ligament between the triquetrum–scaphoid–trapezoid–trapezium (**Fig. 3**). Acknowledging and respecting the architecture of these ligaments during dorsal operative approaches to the wrist helps to maintain the postoperative stability of the wrist.

Superficial Anatomy

Extensor compartments
There are 6 compartments for the wrist extensor tendons on the dorsal and radial wrist. Each compartment is divided by a septum from the extensor retinaculum and contains specific tendons within its sheath. This anatomic arrangement provides a natural series of planes for exposure of the deeper structures. The key landmarks on the extensor side of the wrist are the third compartment, the plane between the second and fourth compartments, the sixth compartment, and the radial border of the fifth compartment. Understanding the anatomy and relationships each of these compartments leads to safer and less traumatic exposures during wrist surgery.

Flexor tendons
The flexor tendons are not contained in discreet retinacular sheaths, as are the extensors.

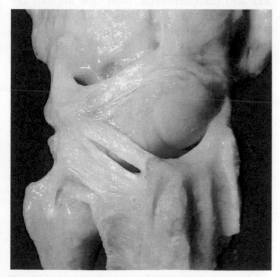

Fig. 3. Cadaveric dissection of the more tenuous dorsal extrinsic ligaments, the dorsal radiotriquetral and intercarpal ligaments. (*Courtesy of* A. Gupta, MD, Louisville, KY.)

Therefore, safely managing the flexor tendons during exposures requires an understanding of the relationships of the tendons to their surrounding structures. The flexor carpi radialis (FCR) flexor carpi ulnaris and the palmaris longus tendons are the most superficial tissues on the volar side of the wrist. Deep to the palmaris longus lies the distal median nerve as it enters the carpal tunnel. Deep to the flexor carpi ulnaris tendon, the ulnar nerve and artery enter Guyon's canal. Deep to the FCR tendon, the radial artery lies proximal to the take-off of the deep palmar branch and the dorsal branch. The digital flexor tendons lie deep to the median nerve at the level of the wrist and superficial to the volar surface of the distal radius and joint capsule of the wrist. Each of these landmarks serves as a locator for the deeper vital structures and allows the surgeon to perform exposures safely by respecting and protecting those structures.

Nerves
The 3 major nerves to the hand—the median, ulnar, and radial nerves—traverse the wrist as they enter the hand. As mentioned, the median and ulnar nerves lie deep to the flexor tendons and are somewhat protected by them during surgical exposures. The radial sensory nerve travels in the superficial subcutaneous plane over the first extensor compartment and radial styloid at the level of the wrist. It branches at the styloid into several distal sensory branches to the dorsal thumb, first webspace, and dorsal index and long fingers (**Fig. 4**). The very superficial location of this nerve and its branches makes it vulnerable to injury during surgical exposure. Likewise, the dorsal sensory branch of the ulnar nerve, which originates from the main trunk of the nerve and travels obliquely and dorsally just distal to the ulnar styloid before branching into several dorsal

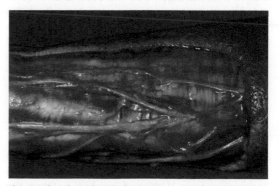

Fig. 4. The dorsal radial sensory nerve lies in the superficial subcutaneous tissues and branches extensively at the level of the distal forearm and wrist. (*Courtesy of* A. Gupta, MD, Louisville, KY.)

cutaneous branches, is vulnerable to injury during surgical exposures on the ulnar side of the wrist. Constant awareness and protection of these superficial nerves during exposures is of critical importance.

STANDARD EXPOSURE OF THE WRIST JOINT

The standard exposure of the wrist joint is used in the treatment of carpal ligament injuries, fractures, and dislocations. This exposure gives excellent visualization of the proximal pole of the scaphoid, but less so the middle and distal bone. It is a dorsal approach through the interval between the second and fourth extensor compartments. The overriding principles of this approach are (a) avoidance of the vulnerable dorsal sensory branches of the radial and ulnar nerves, and (b) maintenance of a synovial sheath around the extensor tendons in the fourth compartment to the fingers, minimizing postoperative scarring and adhesion of the tendons.

The approach is through a midline dorsal incision, centered over Lister's tubercle of the radius and in line with the third ray. Skin flaps are elevated on either side at the level of the extensor retinaculum and can be extended to the mid axial plane on the radial and ulnar borders of the wrist. This elevates the dorsal sensory nerve branches in the skin flaps and protects them from injury. Larger dorsal veins can be elevated in the skin flaps as well, minimizing the need for ligation.

The retinaculum over the third compartment is incised and the extensor pollicis longus tendon is retracted. Continuation of the elevation of the extensor pollicis longus tendon and muscle proximally exposes the posterior interosseous nerve and artery on the dorsal surface of the interosseous membrane. Division of the purely sensory nerve at this level may be performed to create a partial sensory denervation of the wrist for postoperative pain management. The second and fourth extensor compartments are elevated off of the dorsal surface of the radius and capsule of the wrist joint. It is important to maintain the synovial sheath around the fourth compartment tendons as much as possible to maintain a smooth gliding surface for tendon motion and prevent postoperative adhesions to the overlying subcutaneous tissue and the underlying bone and joint capsule.

The joint capsule is incised to expose the underlying distal articular surface of the radius, the radiocarpal joint, and the carpus. A longitudinal incision in line with the third ray or a dorsal ligament-sparing V-shaped incision, splitting the dorsal ligaments parallel to their fibers, rather than sectioning them, can be used to preserve the ligamentous support as much as possible.

At completion of the procedure, closure of the capsule and dorsal ligaments, extensor retinaculum, and skin is performed in a layered fashion in reverse order to the exposure. The extensor pollicis longus tendon can be externalized dorsal to the retinaculum if there is any tension in the dorsal tissue to prevent adhesion or strangulation of the tendon.

STANDARD EXPOSURE OF THE DRUJ

The skin incision for exposure of the DRUJ must respect the underlying dorsal sensory branch of the ulnar nerve. This branch runs obliquely from proximal to distal and volar to dorsal at a roughly 45° angle as it crosses the ulnar head. Thus, the skin incision should be similarly angled to include elevation of this nerve in the skin flap. A longitudinal incision over the dorsal aspect of the distal ulna with a "hockey stick" incision angling radially at the level of the ulnar head, and a zig-zag incision with the radially angled central limb over the ulnar head have both been described.[1]

The extensor retinaculum is separate from the underlying extensor carpi ulnaris sheath and should be elevated as an ulnarly based flap over the extensor carpi ulnaris sheath to prevent disruption of the extensor carpi ulnaris tendon in its anatomic groove over the distal ulna. The retinacular flap incision should start longitudinally over the fifth extensor compartment, with the flap continued obliquely proximally and distally to create the flap. This exposes the dorsal capsule over the DRUJ and the septum between the fourth and fifth compartments. Next, the septum between compartments four and five is elevated off of the DRUJ at the edge of the sigmoid notch and reflected in an ulnar direction. This exposes the DRUJ and TFCC. The ulnar dissection should continue to the edge of the sixth compartment, thus leaving the extensor carpi ulnaris tendon and its sheath in their anatomic location. As the dorsal capsule is elevated from the floor of the fifth compartment in an ulnar direction, it is separated from its attachment to the TFCC immediately volar to it. This allows a direct inspection of the entirety of the TFCC from its radial to its ulnar attachments for direct repair. This exposure gives direct visualization of the DRUJ on both the radial and ulnar sides of the joint. A retractor placed deep to the ulnar head allows the head to be delivered dorsally to better access the full breadth of the sigmoid notch from its dorsal to its volar rim.

A layered repair should be performed at the end of the procedure to restore the structure and support around the DRUJ. Repair of the dorsal ridge of the TFCC to the capsule with mattress sutures insures restoration of dorsal stability. The capsule should be securely reattached to the edge of the fourth–fifth compartment septum on the edge of the radius to reestablish dorsal stability over the distal ulna. Finally, the retinaculum is repaired, completing the exposure.

ALTERNATIVE EXPOSURE OF THE DRUJ

An alternative to the standard exposure to the DRUJ involves raising a radially based retinacular flap from the mid axial line over the ulna to the floor of the fifth compartment. This exposes the underlying extensor carpi ulnaris sheath and tendon directly, and may result in destabilization of the extensor carpi ulnaris tendon if the retinacular dissection is carried too deeply. The remaining exposure of the deeper layers is the same as for the standard approach. Raising the radially based retinacular flap allows use of this flap during closure to create a sling of retinaculum brought around the extensor carpi ulnaris tendon to prevent subluxation of the tendon during forearm rotation (**Fig. 5**). Thus, it may be a more useful exposure in cases where TFCC or DRUJ pathology need to be addressed along with extensor carpi ulnaris sheath disruption and subluxation.

ALTERNATIVE EXPOSURES OF THE WRIST JOINT
Volar Exposure of the Scaphoid

The standard dorsal exposure of the wrist gives excellent exposure of the proximal pole of the scaphoid, extending as far distally as the waist. For exposure of the distal half of the scaphoid and the scaphotrapezial joint, a volar approach is preferred. This gives the surgeon access to the central axis of the scaphoid during open

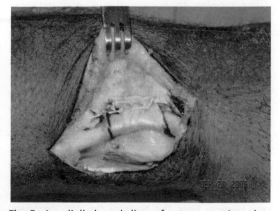

Fig. 5. A radially based sling of extensor retinaculum can be used during closure of the DRUJ exposure to resuspend the extensor carpi ulnaris tendon over the styloid.

compression screw fixation for displaced waist fractures and nonunions. For this approach, the wrist is placed with the palmar side up. A retraction table can be used for stabilization during the initial exposure. A longitudinal incision is made beginning several centimeters proximal to the wrist crease and centered directly over the radial border of the FCR tendon. The longitudinal incision continues to the crease directly over the scaphoid tubercle. Here it is continued at a 45° angle radially and distally over the thenar muscles to the level of the scaphotrapezial joint. The muscle fibers are split along their long axis down to the scaphotrapezial joint capsule. The FCR sheath is incised and the tendon retracted in an ulnar direction, similar to the dissection for volar plating through an FCR incision. The dissection is then brought down across the wrist crease through the dorsal FCR sheath. The tendon is freed distally until it is out of the tunnel in the volar trapezium. The deep volar radial artery and veins send branches across the volar capsule at this level, and these vessels should be ligated to allow access to the volar joint capsule. Deep to the vessels, the radioscaphocapitate ligament is encountered and is divided and identified for later repair during closure. The joint capsule is elevated from the volar scaphoid to the scaphocapitate joint and proximally to the SL ligament to expose the full length of the scaphoid.

To increase the exposure of the bone, the wrist can be extended over a bolster and the wrist fully deviated in an ulnar direction to bring the scaphoid into its elongated position. For screw insertion down the long axis of the scaphoid, the volar rim of the trapezium is dissected away for several millimeters to provide access to the central axis of the scaphoid at its distal articular surface.

In cases of scaphoid nonunion at the waist with humpback collapse, where vascularized bone grafting is planned, a volar corticocancellous graft can be harvested based on perforators from the pronator quadratus muscle. This can be performed simply by extending the incision for the volar exposure of the scaphoid more proximally over the FCR tendon and dissecting the flexor tendons and median nerve off of the pronator quadratus. This allows direct placement of the bone graft into the wedge-shaped defect created by correcting the humpback collapse of the scaphoid with extension of the distal fracture fragment.

DORSAL RADIOCARPAL EXPOSURE FOR VASCULARIZED BONE GRAFTING OF THE SCAPHOID

Vascularized bone grafts from the dorsal surface of the radius are commonly used to treat chronic nonunion and nascent avascular necrosis of the scaphoid, as well as other carpal fractures and avascular necrosis of the lunate, or Kienbock's disease. When addressing nonunions involving the proximal one third of the scaphoid, a dorsal graft is necessary to allow reach of the pedicle to the fracture site and simultaneous exposure of the proximal scaphoid. The most common vascular pedicles used for dorsal bone grafts arise from the dorsal arterial anastomotic network of vessels arising from the dorsal continuation of the anterior interosseous artery after it traverses the interosseous membrane.[2] The 1, 2 intercompartmental supraretinacular artery (ICSRA) is located directly superficial to the retinaculum of the first and second dorsal compartments. The 4 + 5 extensor compartment arterial pedicle is located in the floor of the fourth and fifth compartments deep to the tendons. It lies directly over the periosteal floor of the compartments.

The incision to access the dorsal source vessels, the bone graft sites, and the dorsal scaphoid is a curvilinear incision from the distal forearm dorsal to the interosseous membrane, extending obliquely across the radiocarpal joint line, to the dorsal wrist over the anatomic snuffbox (**Fig. 6**).

When the 1, 2 ICSRA is being used, dissection is carried out carefully in the soft tissues over the retinaculum until the small-caliber vessels (0.5–1.0 mm) are identified, so as not to disrupt the source vessels for the bone graft (**Fig. 7**). The incision is carried out distally to the level of the scaphotrapezial joint capsule. The superficial fascia over the dorsal branch of the radial artery in the snuffbox is carefully incised to expose the vessels. The arterial pedicle for the 1, 2 ICSRA graft is a branch from the radial artery and veins deep to the first compartment tendons. It travels in a dorsovolar direction from the retinaculum to the radial artery. Therefore, once the dorsal pedicle has been identified, the dorsal radiocarpal joint

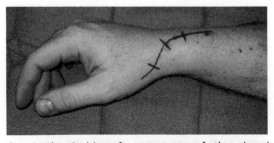

Fig. 6. The incision for exposure of the dorsal scaphoid and donor sites for vascularized bone grafts based on the dorsal arterial anastomotic system begins over the dorsal radial metaphysis in the midline and extends radially in a curved fashion to the dorsal scaphotrapezial joint.

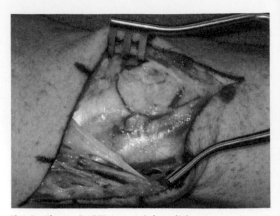

Fig. 7. The 1, 2 ICSRA arterial pedicle.

capsule can be incised from the distal ridge of the radius obliquely over the scaphoid to expose the nonunion site without disrupting the pedicle, which lies proximal to the joint line, deep to the first compartment tendons. Flexion and ulnar deviation of the wrist over a bolster bring the scaphoid into its elongated position and provide better exposure of the proximal pole, the nonunion site, and the remaining scaphoid. The dorsal vessels provide perforators to the dorsal radial bone approximately 1.5 cm proximal to the articular surface of the radius. The bone is exposed by incising the retinaculum on either side of the pedicle and retracting the tendons of the first and second compartment tendons away from the pedicle on either side. This exposes the periosteum over the dorsal radius for harvest of the graft, which can be performed with an oscillating saw and/or osteotomes. The communicating branch between the radial artery and veins and the bone graft can then be dissected from surrounding adventitial tissue to allow rotation of the graft distally to the nonunion site.

The incision to access the 4 + 5 extensor compartment arterial bone graft pedicle is the same as for the 1, 2 ICSRA. The pedicle is found in the floor of the fourth and fifth extensor compartments, deep to the tendons. The retinaculum over the compartments can therefore be incised during the approach, without disrupting the vascular pedicle. The tendons of both compartments are retracted away from each other, exposing the vessels lying on the dorsal periosteum of the radius, as well as the interosseous membrane and the communicating branch between the anterior and posterior interosseous arteries. Ligation of this communicating branch allows extension of a long pedicle from the floor of the fifth compartment, where the bone graft is harvested based on dorsal perforators to the radial cortex, to the floor of the fourth compartment and the dorsal carpal anastomotic vessels, which provide the inflow to the pedicle. This extended pedicle allows the graft to reach the bones of the proximal and distal carpal rows, as well as the base of the metacarpals.

PEARLS AND PITFALLS
Pearls

1. Extensor tendons should be elevated within their synovial compartments, whenever possible, to minimize postoperative scarring and adhesions.
2. The posterior interosseous nerve can be ligated proximal to the wrist joint during dorsal exposures to minimize nociceptive sensory transmission postoperatively, when necessary.
3. Angle the incision for exposure to the DRUJ 45° radially at the ulnar styloid to elevate the dorsal sensory branch of the ulnar nerve in the distal skin flap and prevent injury.
4. Incising the extensor retinaculum and fifth compartment together to elevate tissues off of the DRUJ from radial to ulnar preserves the sheath of the extensor carpi ulnaris tendon and prevents instability and subluxation of the tendon postoperatively.
5. During exposure of the DRUJ, elevation of the capsular flap transversely off of the dorsal limb of the TFCC allows secure reattachment of the TFCC with mattress sutures during closure.
6. Identify and preserve the 2 limbs of the radioscaphocapitate ligament after division during the volar approach to the scaphoid, so that it can be securely repaired with nonabsorbable sutures.
7. Ulnar deviation of the wrist during exposure of the scaphoid from either the volar or dorsal approach brings the bone into its elongated position and allows better visualization of the bone.
8. Resection of the volar rim of the trapezium during open reduction internal fixation of the scaphoid via a volar approach provides access to the central axis of the bone for proper compression screw placement.
9. During harvest of the 1, 2 ICSRA vascularized bone graft from the dorsal radius, elevation and manual compression of the extremity is preferable to Esmarch exsanguination before tourniquet inflation to allow better visualization of the small vessels on the superficial surface of the retinaculum.
10. Use of a volar radial bone graft with perforators from the pronator quadratus muscle allows direct correction of humpback

deformity in treating nonunion of the scaphoid waist. This can be performed through an extension of the standard volar incision for access to the scaphoid.

Pitfalls

1. Avoid exposures that traverse tendon compartments, rather than lie in planes between the compartments, to avoid injury and exposure of the tendons.
2. Elevate sensory nerve branches with skin flaps to avoid nerve injury.
3. Preserve capsular flaps wherever possible during exposure to allow for secure capsular repair to prevent instability.
4. Identify and protect the source vessels during exposure in vascularized bone graft harvest before capsular exposure of the carpus and fracture sites to avoid injury to the pedicle.

CASES
Case 1: Acute SL Ligament Repair via Standard Wrist Exposure

A 48-year-old, right-handed woman presented with an acute SLIL tear after a fall on her dominant right wrist. Radiographs and MRI confirmed wide diastasis between the scaphoid and lunate (**Fig. 8**). The standard dorsal exposure of the wrist was used for repair of the ligament. A straight dorsal incision in line with the third ray was made down to the extensor retinaculum, and the third compartment was incised and the extensor pollicis longus tendon retracted. The second and fourth compartments were elevated off of the underlying wrist capsule, which was incised and reflected to reveal the carpus and the SL joint (**Fig. 9**). Bone anchors were inserted in the proximal scaphoid at the site of ligament detachment

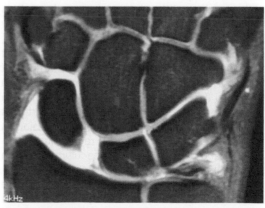

Fig. 8. MRI findings of acute SL dissociation with associated effusion.

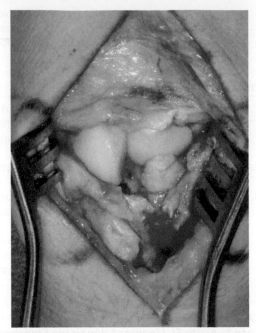

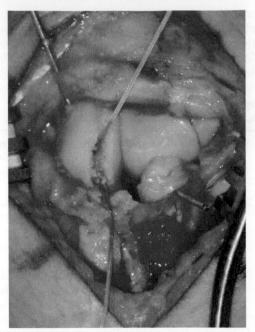

Fig. 9. The standard exposure of the wrist between the second and fourth extensor compartments provides direct access to the scapholunate ligament and mid-carpal row. Note the complete SLIL disruption and wide diastasis.

Fig. 10. Preparation of the SLIL repair with joy sticks in the dorsal scaphoid and lunate and suture anchors inserted in the proximal scaphoid at the site of intended ligament reattachment.

and the sutures passed through the ligament (**Fig. 10**). Joy sticks in the scaphoid and lunate were used to reduce the SL joint, the joint was pinned to maintain reduction during healing, and the ligament was secured to the scaphoid with the suture anchors (**Fig. 11**).

Case 2: Distal Ulna Resection via Standard DRUJ Exposure

An 80-year-old woman presented with chronic instability of the distal ulna and pain after corrective osteotomy for malunion of the radius. A Darrach resection of the distal ulna was planned via the standard exposure of the DRUJ. A hockey stick incision was made over the distal ulna, continuing distally with a 45° radial extension at the ulnar styloid (**Fig. 12**). The dorsal branch of the ulnar nerve was identified in and elevated in the distal flap for protection (**Fig. 13**). An incision was made over the fifth extensor compartment down to the tendon, with a distal extension in line with the fibers of the dorsal radiotriquetral ligament, and the extensor retinaculum and fifth compartment sheath were elevated from the sigmoid notch ulnarly to the level of the sixth compartment. The extensor carpi ulnaris tendon was left undisturbed in its sheath to prevent instability and subluxation (**Fig. 14**). This exposed the

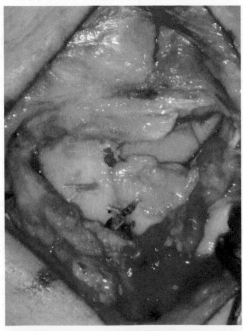

Fig. 11. Final repair of acute complete SLIL tear with correction of diastasis and reattachment of the SLIL to the proximal scaphoid via suture anchors.

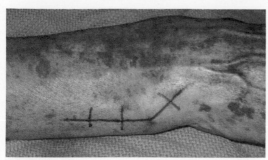

Fig. 12. The standard incision for exposure of the DRUJ. The incision should be angled at 45° radially at the ulnar styloid to protect the dorsal branch of the ulnar nerve.

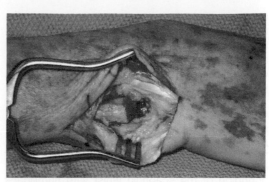

Fig. 15. Completion of resection of the distal ulna to the level of the proximal sigmoid notch. Note the extensor carpi ulnaris tendon remains entirely contained in its sheath.

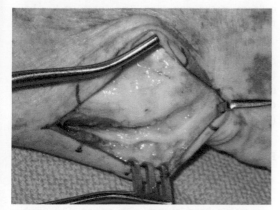

Fig. 13. The dorsal ulnar sensory nerve elevated in the distal skin flap.

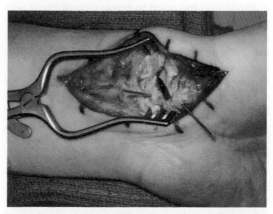

Fig. 16. The volar exposure of the scaphoid. The nonunion has been exposed and joy sticks placed in the proximal and distal fragments for manipulation and preparation of the bone for graft placement.

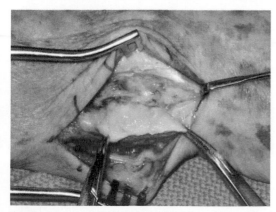

Fig. 14. The dorsal retinacular flap with the roof of the fifth compartment elevated and reflected (hemostats) to show the underlying dorsal capsule over the DRUJ.

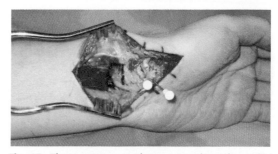

Fig. 17. The pronator quadratus over the volar radial cortex provides a rich source of perforators for vascularized bone grafting of the scaphoid. The muscle and bone can be exposed by extending the volar scaphoid incision proximally.

ulnar head, which was resected with a rongeur to the level of the proximal sigmoid notch (**Fig. 15**). Layered closure repaired the joint capsule and the juncture of the fourth and fifth compartments, without disruption of the extensor carpi ulnaris tendon sheath.

Case 3: Vascularized Radial Bone Graft Reconstruction of Scaphoid Nonunion via Extended Volar Approach

A 26-year-old man presented with a chronic nonunion of the scaphoid waist with humpback collapse. Reconstruction was approached through the volar exposure of the scaphoid. A V-shaped, longitudinal incision was made across the wrist crease at the radial border of the FCR tendon, extending distally to the level of the scaphotrapezial joint. Because of the humpback collapse and the need to correct longitudinal and volar deficiency in the scaphoid, the incision was extended to the level of the proximal aspect of the pronator quadratus. The radiscaphocapitate ligament was divided and identified for repair during closure, as well as the volar joint capsule. The nonunion site was exposed and joy sticks placed in the fragments for manipulation of the proximal and distal bone (**Fig. 16**). The devitalized bone was resected and the size of the graft determined by extending the scaphoid into its fully upright position using the joy sticks. The pronator quadratus was exposed and the flap outlined on the muscle, centered over the radial cortex 1.5 cm proximal to the radiocarpal joint, with visualization of the intramuscular perforators confirming the site of the pedicle (**Fig. 17**). The graft was then harvested using an oscillating saw, taking care to keep the muscle and periosteum intact over the volar cortex

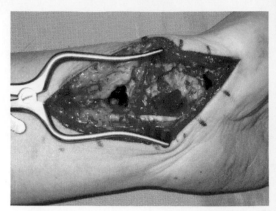

Fig. 18. The graft has been inset into the scaphoid defect. Note the cancellous block has been contoured to the dimensions of the upright scaphoid, and the radial cortex with pronator quadratus muscle restores volar cortical integrity and corrects the previous volar collapse at the nonunion. The construct has been fixed with a longitudinal compression screw.

of the graft. The graft was then securely inset into the defect in the scaphoid and the scaphoid–graft–scaphoid construct fixed with a longitudinal compression screw under fluoroscopic guidance (**Fig. 18**).

REFERENCES

1. Garcia-Elias M. Carpal instability. In: Wolfe SW, Hotchkiss RN, Pederson WC, et al, editors. Green's operative hand surgery. 6th edition. Philadelphia: Elsevier Churchill Livingstone; 2011. p. 465–522.
2. Zaidemberg C, Siebert JW, Angrigiani C. A new vascularized bone graft for scaphoid nonunion. J Hand Surg 1991;16A:474–8.

Surgical Exposures of the Hand

Andrew J. Watt, MD[a,b,*], Kevin C. Chung, MD, MS[c]

KEYWORDS

- Metacarpal • Phalanx • Hand trauma • Approach • Exposure

KEY POINTS

- Surgical approaches to the hand are designed to correct injury or deformity with minimal morbidity.
- Useful surgical approaches are versatile, safe, preserve critical structures, and have an acceptable aesthetic outcome.
- Choice of an appropriate surgical approach requires a detailed understanding of normal and structural pathology.
- Dorsal approaches are common and are generally safe.
- Volar approaches allow for fixation in a specialized subset of injuries including intraarticular injuries.

INTRODUCTION

Choosing the appropriate surgical approach to any structure in the hand requires a detailed understanding of the normal anatomy and the structural pathology associated with the particular injury or disease process being treated. The goal of any surgical approach is simple: To correct deformity or injury while avoiding morbidity. Execution, however, remains more complex. Any surgical approach to the hand should be versatile, providing sufficient exposure of the structures requiring repair. It should also provide the ability to expand the exposure proximally and distally to introduce necessary devices for fixation. In addition to versatility, surgical exposures should be safe. Critical structures should be easily identified, preserved, and reconstructed. Surgical exposures should also preserve inherent stability and strength of the tendons and ligamentous structures of the hand. Consideration should also be given to the functional and aesthetic units of the hand and the resultant scar.

We have reviewed pertinent hand anatomy and common surgical approaches to the hand, with a principal focus on treatment of metacarpal and phalangeal injuries. Each surgical approach is evaluated with respect to the core principles of versatility, safety, preservation of stability, and aesthetics.

ANATOMY OF THE HAND AND DIGITS

Knowledge of the cutaneous, osseous, ligamentous, musculotendinous, vascular, and nerve anatomy of the hand is an essential prerequisite for designing and performing surgical approaches in the hand.

Cutaneous Anatomy

The cutaneous envelope of the hand is highly specialized, reflecting both structure and function. The dorsal skin of the hand is thin and pliable, allowing for nearly unrestricted motion. Landmarks including the extensor tendons and bony

Funding Sources: No funding sources to disclose.

Conflict of Interest: No conflict of interest to disclose.

[a] Department of Plastic Surgery, The Buncke Clinic, California Pacific Medical Center, 45 Castro Street, Suite 121, San Francisco, CA 94114, USA; [b] Division of Plastic and Reconstructive Surgery, Stanford University School of Medicine, 770 Welch Road, Suite 400, Stanford, CA 94304, USA; [c] Department of Surgery, University of Michigan Medical School, 2130 Taubman Center, 1500 East Medical Center Drive, Ann Arbor, MI 48109, USA

* Corresponding author. The Buncke Clinic, 45 Castro Street, Suite 121, San Francisco, CA 94114.

E-mail address: ajwatt50@gmail.com

structures may be easily palpated dorsally. The skin of the palm is glabrous and devoid of hair follicles, with a thickened dermal component. The skin of the palm is durable and has a unique capacity for robust secondary wound healing.[1]

Osseous and Ligametous Anatomy

The bony anatomy of the metacarpals and phalanges takes origin from the distal carpal row. The distal carpal row forms a solid architectural arch with the capitate as its keystone.[2] This fixed transverse arch is carried distally to the more mobile adaptive transverse arch of the metacarpal heads and is complemented by the volar convexity of the metacarpals. This anatomy ensures that the palm is convex in both the proximal–distal and radial–ulnar dimensions, which allow the palm to hold convex objects.

With the exception of the thumb carpometacarpal (CMC) joint, the CMC joints of the fingers are relatively immobile. Mobility increases ulnarly with the index and long fingers nearly fixed whereas the ring and small finger exhibit a 15° to 25° arc of flexion–extension.[3] The thumb CMC is unique as a biconcave–convex saddle joint that imparts versatile cone of thumb motion. The metacarpophalangeal (MCP) joints afford significantly more mobility. These joints are condyloid, allowing not only flexion and extension but radial and ulnar deviation (abduction and adduction). Radial and ulnar motion at the MCP is stabilized by collateral ligaments. Because of the cam structure of the MCP joint, these ligaments are lax with the MCP in extension and taught with the MCP in flexion. The net effect is that the MCP is more stable in flexion during lateral pinch.[4] Although the collateral ligaments constrain lateral displacement, the firm volar plate resists hyperextension, and the intervening extensions between the volar plate—the intermetacarpal ligament—stabilizes the distal metacarpal arch.

The thumb consists of a proximal and distal phalanx, whereas the index, long, ring, and small fingers are composed of 3 phalanges. Each interphalangeal joint is stabilized against radial- and ulnar-directed stress with proper and accessory radial and ulnar collateral ligaments (UCLs). Stout volar plates prevent hyperextension at the proximal interphalangeal (PIP) joint level and to a lesser degree at the distal interphalangeal (DIP) joint level. The UCL of the thumb is of particular clinical relevance because it is prone to both acute disruption (skier's thumb) and chronic attenuation (gamekeeper's thumb). The proper UCL of the thumb stabilizes the thumb MCP joint against radially directed forces such as those generated in pinch activities with the MCP in slight flexion whereas the accessory collateral ligament and volar plate contribute to stability in full MCP extension.

Musculotendinous Anatomy

The musculotendinous structure of the hand relies on the balanced coordination of extrinsic and intrinsic structures. The thumb is powered extrinsically by the extensor pollicis longus (EPL) and flexor pollicis longus. The EPL traverses the wrist in the third dorsal compartment, inserting onto the base of the distal phalanx. In its course, the EPL tendon forms the dorsal–ulnar border to the anatomic snuff box. The flexor pollicis longus tendon travels through the carpal tunnel and travels via a stout fibroosseous canal to insert on the volar base of the distal phalanx. The abductor pollicis longus (APL) and extensor pollicis brevis (EPB) serve as additional extrinsic movers of the thumb. At the level of the wrist, the APL and EPB tendons traverse the first dorsal compartment and insert on the bases of the thumb metacarpal and proximal phalanx, respectively. In this course, they form the radial–volar border of the anatomic snuff box, a critical landmark; the dorsal branch of the radial artery traverses this interval. The intrinsic musculature of the thumb consists of the abductor pollicis brevis, flexor pollicis brevis, and opponens pollicis. These musculotendinous units act primarily across the CMC joint, allowing for abduction, flexion, and opposition of the thumb. The small finger maintains analogous abductor, flexor, and opponens muscles comprising the hypothenar musculature.

The index, long, ring, and small fingers are similarly powered both by intrinsic and extrinsic musculotendinous units. The extensor digitorum communis (EDC) powers each finger via a common extrinsic muscle belly. These tendons contribute to the complexity of the dorsal extensor apparatus of the finger. The tendons emerge from the fourth dorsal compartment and are centralized over the MCP joints by radial and ulnar sagittal bands. Over the proximal phalanx, the extensor tendon becomes broad, receiving contributions from the intrinsic interossei and lumbricals. These contributions create the well-defined lateral bands of the extensor mechanism. The central substance of the extensor hood terminates via insertion into the base of the middle phalanx. The lateral bands continue distally to insert onto the dorsal base of the distal phalanx. The index and small fingers have additional proper extensor tendons (extensor indicis proprius and extensor digiti minimi) that travel ulnar and just deep to their EDC counterparts. These tendons serve to independently extend the index and small fingers. Junturae tendinae serve as intertendinous connections over the dorsum of the hand, further interconnecting the common extensor tendons. The flexor mechanism of the fingers is equally complex. Flexor digitiorum superficialis (FDS) and profundus (FDP) tendons traverse the carpal tunnel and enter the fibroosseous canal of the fingers consisting of 5 annular and 3 cruciate pulleys. The FDS tendons lie volar to the FDP tendons until they diverge at Camper's chiasm and each slip of the FDS tendon turns 180° to insert onto the middle phalanx. The FDS tendons, therefore, primarily serve to flex the PIP joints. The FDP tendon continues distally to insert at the base of the distal phalanx serving to flex both the PIP and DIP joints.

The intrinsic muscles of the hand consist of the interossei and lumbricals. The interossei occupy the space between the metacarpals. The dorsal interossei serve to abduct the fingers and the volar interossei serve to adduct the fingers. The first dorsal interosseous muscle is unique in taking origin from the thumb metacarpal and inserting into the extensor expansion of the index finger. This muscle serves to abduct the index finger while adducting the thumb, making it an integral component of power pinch. In addition to the interossei, 4 lumbrical muscles take origin from the FDP tendon and insert into the radial aspect of the extensor hood. These unique muscles lie volar to the axis of rotation of the MCP joint and dorsal to the axis of rotation of the PIP joints, serving to flex the MCP and extend the PIP joints.

Vascular Anatomy

The arterial supply to the hand is robust and highly interconnected. Arterial supply is via the radial and ulnar arteries. The radial artery bifurcates at the level of the radial styloid and sends a dominant dorsal branch through the floor of the anatomic snuff box. The dorsal branch of the radial artery traverses the first dorsal interosseous muscle passing dorsal to volar and becoming the principal contributor to the deep palmar arch and the princeps pollicis artery. The princeps pollicis subsequently gives rise to the proper radial and ulnar digital arteries to the thumb as well as the radial digital artery to the index finger. The volar branch of the radial artery joins the ulnar artery via the superficial palmar arch. The ulnar artery bifurcates at the level of the wrist, sending a minor contribution to the deep palmar arch and a major contribution to the superficial palmar arch. At the mid metacarpal level, the superficial palmar arch gives rise

to common digital arteries to the second, third, and fourth web spaces. These common digital arteries bifurcate at the level of the MCP joint into proper digital arteries. These arteries further divide at the distal phalanx, trifurcating into a pulp vessel, a paronychial branch, and a dorsal branch to supply the finger tip. The proper digital arteries accompany the proper digital nerves in the finger, volar to the mid axis of the finger. Collateral flow also occurs via interconnections between the common and proper digital arteries in the palm and finger. In addition to the dominant palmar circulation to the hand, a dorsal circulation exists based on the dorsal carpal branches of the radial and ulnar arteries. These arteries give rise to the dorsal metacarpal arteries that lie deep to the fascia, in the interosseous space. The dorsal circulation communicates with the volar circulation via perforating arteries in the web spaces.

Although volar veins exist in the hand, the predominant venous drainage of the hand is dorsal. Dorsal digital veins coalesce to form dorsal veins of the hand and ultimately drain via the cephalic and basilic veins.

Nerve Anatomy

The hand is innervated by the radial, median, and ulnar nerves. The radial nerve contribution to the hand is entirely sensory, providing innervation of the dorsal–radial aspect of the hand. The superficial branch of the radial nerve arises from its course deep to the brachioradialis approximately 5 cm proximal to the radial styloid, sending 3 to 5 branches to the dorsal hand.[2,5] These branches transmit sensory information form the dorsal aspect of the thumb, index, long, and radial half of the ring finger from the level of the DIP joint proximally.

The median nerve enters the hand via the carpal tunnel. The radial, volar portion of the median nerve gives off the recurrent motor branch to the thenar musculature. A number of clinically pertinent variations of recurrent motor branch anatomy have been described, including subligamentous and transligamentous branching patterns, as well as abnormal origin from the ulnar aspect of the median nerve.[6] Beyond this point, the median nerve innervates the 2 most radial lumbricals and then becomes entirely sensory by giving rise to common digital nerves to the first, second, and third web spaces. The proper digital nerve to the thumb arises at the distal metacarpal level and the radial digital nerve to the thumb that typically crosses over or just proximal to the A-1 pulley of the thumb. The common digital nerves lie dorsal to the common digital arteries in the palm. This relationship becomes inverted as both the nerves and arteries divide into their proper terminal components with the proper digital nerve lying volar to the proper digital arteries in the fingers.

The ulnar nerve enters the hand via the Guyon canal, radial to the pisiform and ulnar to the hook of the hamate. The ulnar nerve divides into a deep motor branch and a superficial sensory branch. The deep motor branch innervates the hypothenar musculature, dorsal and palmar interossei, the ulnar 2 lumbricals, the adductor pollicis, and the deep head of the flexor pollicis brevis. The superficial sensory component gives rise to the common digital nerve to the fourth web space as well as the proper digital nerve to the ulnar aspect of the small finger. The ulnar nerve also provides sensory innervation for the dorsal–ulnar aspect of the hand with 1 to 2 cutaneous branches. These branches transmit sensory information from the small and ulnar half of the ring finger from the level of the DIP joint proximally.

FUNCTIONAL AESTHETIC SUBUNITS OF THE HAND

The application of the aesthetic subunit concept has been espoused in nasal, breast, and foot and ankle reconstruction.[7–9] Although reconstructive hand surgeons have informally applied these principles to reconstruction of the hand, the

division of the hand into characteristic regions of narrowing, curvature, and projection has been more recently discussed in a more organized fashion.[10] Topographic contrast with regions of convexity and concavity divided by skin creases separate the hand into seven distinct subunits: (1) Thenar (T), (2) hypothenar (H), (3) central triangle (C), (4) opposition (O), (5) metacarpal area (M), (6) dorsal hand (D), (7) Volar and dorsal surfaces of the fingers as well as pulp (P) and nail unit (N; **Fig. 1**). These subunits also echo underlying functional units of the hand. Because of that special relationship between function and aesthetics of the hand, Abdel-Rehim and colleagues[10] coined the term "functional aesthetic units and subunits" of the hand. When possible, one should place skin incisions in the intervals between these subunits, rather than crossing subunits. Respecting these subunits improves the cosmetic outcomes.

METACARPAL EXPOSURES

Surgical approaches to the metacarpals are generally employed in the fixation of fractures and, less commonly, in the treatment of bony deformities and tumors. These approaches are commonly placed on the dorsal aspect of the hand. Volar approaches contend with critical neurovascular structures, including the superficial and

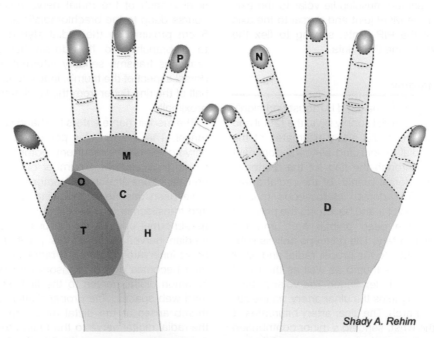

Shady A. Rehim

Fig. 1. Functional aesthetic units and subunits of the hand: Thenar (T), hypothenar (H), central triangle (C), opposition (O), metacarpal area (M), dorsal hand (D), volar and dorsal surfaces of the fingers as well as pulp (P) and nail unit (N). (*Courtesy of* Dr S.A. Rehim, MB ChB, MSc, Ann Arbor, MI.)

deep palmar arch, as well as the median nerve, recurrent motor branch to the thumb, and deep motor contributions of the ulnar nerve. The volar anatomy is in distinct contrast with the reliably safe exposure over the dorsal anatomy containing the dorsal veins, dorsal cutaneous branches of the radial and ulnar nerves, and the extensor tendons.

Index, Long, Ring, and Small Finger Metacarpals

The metacarpal base, diaphysis, and head may all be approached via axial incisions placed on the dorsum of the hand (**Fig. 2**). These approaches are safe, and may easily be extended proximally and distally to improve exposure. The location on the dorsum of the hand is not cosmetically favorable. To achieve good scar appearance, one should minimize the length of the incision and force of retraction.

Metacarpal base

The metacarpal base requires exposure in cases of intraarticular fractures and irreducible dislocations. A 1.5- to 2-cm incision is centered directly over the metacarpal base, which is typically palpable (see **Fig. 2**A.6). In the case of substantial edema, fluoroscopic guidance may be useful in planning incision placement. Once the skin in incised, longitudinal spreads with tenotomy or Littler scissors helps to identify any subcutaneous veins and dorsal cutaneous nerves. Transverse veins may be ligated with surgical clips while preserving the longitudinal veins. The cutaneous nerve should be mobilized and retracted. The dorsal capsule of the CMC joints is divided longitudinally to expose the joint and the metacarpal base. The second and third metacarpal bases serve as the point of insertion for the extensor carpi radialis longus and extensor carpi radialis brevus tendons, respectively, whereas the fifth metacarpal base serves as the point of

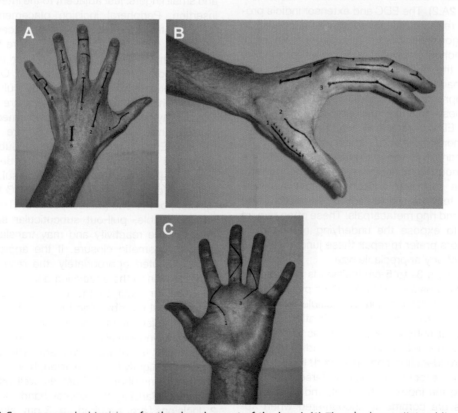

Fig. 2. (*A*) Common surgical incisions for the dorsal aspect of the hand. (1) Thumb ulnar collateral ligament. (2) Metacarpal. (3) Proximal phalanx. (4) Metacarpophalangeal joint (metacarpal head and proximal phalangeal base). (5) Distal interphalangeal joint. (6) Metacarpal base. (7) Middle phalanx. (8) Proximal interphalangeal joint. (*B*) Common surgical incisions for the lateral aspect of the hand. (1) Thumb metacarpophalangeal joint via EPL/EPB interval (adjacent *dotted line* indicates trans EPL approach). (2) Thumb ulnar collateral ligament. (3) Midaxial incision, proximal phalanx, collateral ligament, and middle phalanx. (4) Midaxial incision translated distally. (*C*) Common surgical incisions for the volar aspect of the hand. (1) Metacarpal head and neck. (2) Proximal interphalangeal joint (proximal phalangeal head and middle phalangeal base). (3) Metacarpophalangeal joint (metacarpal head and proximal phalangeal base).

insertion for the extensor carpi ulnaris tendon. These tendon insertions may be divided longitudinally while preserving their periosteal attachment or disinserted. If the tendon is disinserted, it should be repaired.

Metacarpal diaphysis

Approach to the metacarpal diaphysis is among the most facile and common approaches to the hand. This approach is used for the open treatment of metacarpal fractures. The index and long finger metacarpals lie just radial to their associated EDC tendons. The ring finger metacarpal lies directly beneath its EDC tendon, whereas the small finger metacarpal lies just ulnar to its associated EDC tendon and directly beneath the EDM. Knowledge of relative position of the extensor tendon to the underlying bone facilitates the exposure. The index finger metacarpal is best exposed via a longitudinal incision placed directly over the metacarpal, radial to the extensor mechanism (see **Fig. 2**A.2). The EDC and extensor indicis proprius are retracted ulnarly to provide exposure. In an analogous fashion, the long finger metacarpal is approached just radial to the extensor tendon, whereas the ring and small finger metacarpals are approached just ulnar to the extensor tendon. When approaching the small finger, the surgeon may choose to enter the interval between the EDC and EDM or remain ulnar to the EDM. The authors generally prefer to remain ulnar to the EDM by retracting this tendon radially along with the EDC without violating the extensor mechanism. Juncturae may be encountered between the extensor tendons, particularly when approaching the long and ring metacarpals. These often require division to expose the underlying metacarpals. The authors prefer to repair these juncturae when they are of any appreciable size.

Generally, a 3- to 5-cm incision is required for sufficient exposure and to introduce plate fixation; a slightly smaller incision is possible when performing interfragmentary screw fixation (**Fig. 3**). Longitudinal subcutaneous veins as well as the cutaneous nerve branches of the radial and ulnar nerves are identified and preserved. Radial nerve branches are commonly encountered when approaching the index metacarpal, and ulnar nerve branches are commonly encountered when approaching the small finger metacarpal. Nerve branches are often absent or diminutive in the central portion of the hand when approaching the long and ring finger metacarpals.

The dorsum of each metacarpal has a characteristic "bare area" that lies between the interosseous muscles and is covered only by periosteum. Periosteal incision and elevation must be sufficient

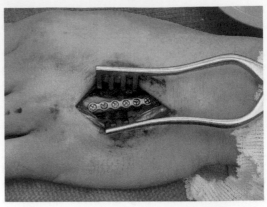

Fig. 3. Dorsal metacarpal diaphyseal exposure.

for fracture reduction and for placement of hardware. The periosteal incision is placed radial on the index and long fingers and ulnar on the ring and small fingers, just adjacent to the interosseous insertion. Peripheral incision placement allows for potential coverage of the metacarpal and implanted hardware. Periosteal closure is undertaken with interrupted figure of 8 or a running 4-O Monocryl (Ethicon, Cincinnati, OH, USA) suture. Periosteal closure is often difficult, particularly in when multiple metacarpals are fracture. Repair may be left loose or not performed without consequence. Divided juncturae are repaired with 4-O Ethibond (Ethicon) sutures. Subcuticular closure is accomplished with deep dermal 4-0 Monocryl (Ethicon) sutures, whereas subcuticular closure is completed with a running 4-O Monocryl (Ethicon) or Prolene (Ethicon) suture. The use of a nonabsorbable, pull-out subcuticular suture reduces tissue reactivity and may translate into a superior cosmetic closure. If the approach has been executed appropriately, the resultant scar from the skin to the underlying periosteum should be radial or ulnar to the extensor mechanism, reducing but not obviating tendon adhesion.

When adjacent metacarpals require operative fixation, a single incision placed in the interval between the 2 metacarpals is made. This approach requires a slightly longer incision; however, it minimizes the number of scars as well as the risk of devascularizing the dorsal hand skin. When 2 incisions are required, a 3-cm skin bridge between the incisions should be preserved. The intervening skin acts as a bipedicled flap and should be handled meticulously to avoid tissue necrosis.

Metacarpal head and neck

The metacarpal head and neck necessitate exposure in cases of displaced intraarticular fractures, irreducible MCP joint dislocations, and rarely in the case of an irreducible metacarpal neck fracture. At this level both dorsal and volar approaches are possible (see **Fig. 2**A.4, C.1).

The dorsal approach remains facile, safe, and affords minimal destabilization. The dorsal cutaneous branches of the radial and ulnar nerve are diminutive and do not factor substantially into the approach. The extensor mechanism and the relationship to the radial and ulnar sagittal bands are a concern at this level because these structures lie directly over the metacarpal head. Access to the metacarpal head may be obtained by 1 of 2 methods: Division of the sagittal band with subsequent repair or a longitudinal split of the extensor mechanism.

The extensor mechanism exerts an ulnar vector of pull across the MCP joint; consequently, the extensor tendon tends to sublux ulnarly in the absence of a stout radial sagittal band. With this consideration in mind, the ulnar sagittal band is preferentially divided to reduce the risk of postoperative extensor subluxation. Leaving a cuff of longitudinal fibers of the central portion of the extensor tendon with the ulnar sagittal band facilitates repair. When sutures are placed during the repair, they are perpendicular to these longitudinal fibers rather than parallel and this simple variation in technique lends strength to the repair.

A true longitudinal split of the extensor mechanism is facile and obviates the issue of postoperative tendon subluxation. This split is carried out in the direction of the longitudinal fibers within the central substance of the tendon. Single skin hooks may be used to place the tendon on tension and a no. 15 blade is used to make the longitudinal incision. The dorsal joint capsule comes into view and is divided longitudinally to access the articular surface of the metacarpal head or the joint itself in cases of irreducible dislocations.

This approach is most commonly used in the treatment of irreducible MCP dislocations where the volar plate is interposed, dorsal to the metacarpal head.[11–16] In this instance, the volar plate comes into view once the central portion of the extensor tendon is split. The volar plate typically requires partial longitudinal division to facilitate reduction (**Fig. 4**). Advocates of the dorsal approach to MCP reduction cite relative safety compared with the volar approach, as well as ease of dissection.[11–14,17]

The MCP joint may be approached from the volar aspect of the hand as well. This approach is primarily employed in the treatment of irreducible MCP dislocations and may be extended distally to approach proximal phalangeal base fractures.[16,18–20] The volar MCP approach is designed as a Bruner incision centered over the MCP joint and may be extended proximally or distally as necessitated by the underlying pathology. The skin is incised and the radial and ulnar neurovascular bundles are identified and preserved. These bundles may be displaced superficially in cases of MCP dislocation, and should be identified first. The A-1 pulley and the flexor tendon sheath are divided longitudinally; the A-2 pulley is preserved, and the flexor tendons are retracted to expose the underlying volar plate. To gain access to the MCP joint, the volar plate may be divided proximally from the metacarpal. Neither the A-1 pulley nor the volar plate require repair.

Thumb Metacarpal

Metacarpal base

The anatomy and approach to the thumb metacarpal is unique. Accurate reduction of thumb metacarpal base fractures is critical in preserving the thumb CMC joint surface and often require an incision. The thumb metacarpal base may be approached dorsally just radial to the EPL tendon.

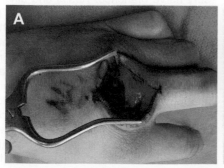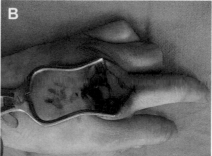

Fig. 4. Dorsal metacarpophalangeal dislocation. (*A*) Ulnar sagittal band divided, extensor tendon retracted radially. (*B*) after partial division of volar plate and reduction.

Generally, a 2-cm incision is placed directly over the metacarpal base. Dorsal cutaneous branches of the radial nerve as well as cutaneous veins are preserved. The dorsal branch of the radial artery crosses over the scaphotrapezial interval and must be identified, dissected free, and retracted ulnarly. The APL tendon inserts onto the base of the metacarpal and is elevated in conjunction with the periosteum. This approach provides excellent exposure of the dorsal metacarpal base as well as the radial condyle of the metacarpal; however, access to the volar ulnar metacarpal Bennett's fracture fragment is limited.

The volar aspect of the metacarpal base is more easily visualized via a Wagner approach. The Wagner incision is placed at the junction of the glabrous and dorsal skin of the hand. The longitudinal limb is designed over the subcutaneous border of the metacarpal in the interval between the APL and thenar musculature. Proximally, the incision follows the thenar musculature toward the radial border of the flexor carpi radialis tendon. The palmar cutaneous branch of the median nerve lies just ulnar to the FCR tendon and is protected so long as the dissection does not proceed ulnarly. The thenar musculature is elevated in a subperiosteal plane and the joint capsule is incised to expose the metacarpal base. This incision in particularly favorable from a cosmetic standpoint as the scar lies in the transition between the glabrous and nonglabrous skin. The periosteum is repaired with 4-O PDS (Ethicon) suture to restore the muscle origin. The skin may be closed with cuticular or a subcuticular suture.

Metacarpal diaphysis

Analogous to surgical approaches to the non-thumb metacarpals, surgical exposure of the thumb metacarpal is primarily accomplished via a dorsal approach. A 2- to 3-cm incision is placed in the interval between the EPL and EPB tendons. At the level of the MCP, the EPL and EPB tendons share a common extensor expansion with radial and ulnar sagittal bands. The vector of the EPL tendon favors ulnar subluxation in cases of instability; therefore, if the dissection requires distal extension, the ulnar sagittal band should be preferentially divided.

Metacarpal head

Access to the metacarpal head and MCP joint are required in instances of MCP dislocation, intraarticular fractures and in UCL injuries. The standard dorsal approach to the thumb MCP is centered over the joint in the interval between the EPL and EPB (see **Fig. 2**B.1). A 2- to 3-cm skin incision is made and subcutaneous flaps are elevated

radially and ulnarly. The interval between the EPL and EPB is sharply incised, as is the dorsal joint capsule. The EPB insertion into the base of the proximal phalanx is elevated with the radial periosteal flap. Closure is accomplished by reapproximating the EPL–EPB interval the level of the MCP.

Alternatively, the metacarpal head and MCP joint can be accessed through a trans-EPL approach. This approach affords facile access to the MCP joint in cases of intraarticular metacarpal head fractures and irreducible MCP dislocations and preserves stability of the extensor mechanism at the MCP joint level. The skin incision is placed directly over the EPL tendon at the level of the MCP joint. The skin is sharply incised and radial and ulnar skin flaps are elevated to expose the EPL tendon. The tendon is then incised sharply in line with its fibers, splitting the tendon along its proximal–distal course. The dorsal joint capsule is then incised to gain access to the joint. The EPL tendon is then closed longitudinally with a running 4-O clear nylon or Prolene suture (Ethicon). The EPL excursion is ensured postoperatively by allowing for motion at the interphalangeal joint of the thumb to avoid tendon adhesion.

UCL

Repair of the UCL is commonly performed. The UCL complex arises from the ulnar collateral recess of the thumb metacarpal head. The proper collateral ligament arises dorsally within the collateral recess and travels obliquely to insert on the volar one third of the proximal phalangeal base. Surgical approach to the UCL is undertaken in cases of complete disruption of the UCL. Surgical approach is designed as a 2- to 3-cm linear or curvilinear incision centered over the ulnar border of the thumb MCP joint (see **Fig. 2**B.2). The distal limb of the incision falls in line with the mid axis of the thumb. The skin is sharply incised. Longitudinal spreads are used to identify any terminal sensory nerve branches. Radial and ulnar skin flaps are elevated in the loose aponeurotic plane. The adductor aponeurosis and radial sagittal band is divided to enter the collateral ligament complex, leaving a 1- to 2-mm cuff of tissue radially for repair. In cases of complete collateral ligament avulsion from the proximal phalangeal base, the ligament often lies dorsal to the adductor aponeurosis and should be identified before dividing the aponeurosis. After ligament repair, the adductor aponeurosis is repaired with 4-0 PDS (Ethicon) or Vicryl (Ethicon) suture, taking care not to incorporate the EPL tendon into the repair. The skin is then closed with 4-O Monocryl (Ethicon) deep dermal sutures and subcuticular closure accomplished with 4-O Monocryl (Ethicon) or 4-O Prolene (Ethicon) as a pull-out suture. Despite being on the dorsal aspect of the hand, this incision has a good appearance because it is hidden within the skin creases of the first web space at the junction of the glabrous and nonglabrous skin.[21–23]

PROXIMAL PHALANGEAL EXPOSURES

Surgical exposure to the proximal phalanx is undertaken primarily to fix unstable fractures and intraarticular fractures of the proximal phalanx. Because of the intimate relation between the extensor mechanism and the underlying bone, prevention of postoperative stiffness and adhesion is a primary consideration.

Index, Long, Ring, and Small Finger Proximal Phalanges

Dorsal, lateral, and volar approaches provide exposure for the treatment of proximal phalangeal fractures and for the resection of bony tumors. The dorsal approach is technically simple and affords the ability to extend the approach proximally and distally (see **Fig. 2**A.3). The dorsal extensor apparatus at this level consists of the central tendon that terminally inserts onto the base of the middle phalanx and the lateral bands that drape over the lateral surface of the proximal phalanx. The dorsal approach is a distal extension of the approach described for the metacarpal head and proximal phalangeal base. The incision is centered over the central tendon. At this level, dorsal veins are the only relevant intervening structure between the skin and underlying tendon. Radial and ulnar skin flaps are raised and the central tendon is splint longitudinally, preserving the terminal insertion into the base of the middle phalanx. The periosteum is then incised and elevated off of the underlying bone. The longitudinal tendon split is closed with 4-O clear nylon or PDS (Ethicon) suture. Skin closure is accomplished with deep dermal 4-O Monocryl (Ethicon) sutures and a running subcuticular 5-O Monocryl (Ethicon) or pull-out Prolene (Ethicon) suture.[23–25] Alternatively, the proximal phalanx and PIP joint may be exposed via a Chamay approach through the extensor tendon. The cutaneous incision remains identical to that previously described; however, the central portion of the extensor tendon is elevated as a distally based triangular flap, leaving the lateral bands intact.[26] This exposure provides direct access to the dorsal aspect of the proximal phalanx and the PIP joint. Repair of the tendon flap is performed with interrupted 4-O nylon or Eithibond (Ethicon) sutures. Interrupted sutures

are preferred in this repair to distribute the load when motion is started.

Given the diminutive size of the proximal phalanx and intimate association of the extensor tendon with the underlying bone, hardware placement is often challenging to prevent tendon adhesions. These factors favor lateral hardware placement. A mid axial approach allows for expansile exposure of the phalanx (see **Fig. 2**B.3). The incision is designed along points connecting the axis of rotation of the MCP, PIP, and DIP joints. These points can be approximated by placing the finger in flexion and marking the dorsal aspect of the resultant PIP and DIP skin creases. A skin incision may be placed at any point along this line and is easily customized to accommodate the underlying pathology and any implants that require placement. Appropriate incision design places the neurovascular bundles volar to the planned incision. A single dorsal cutaneous branch of the proper digital nerve typically traverses the approach at the junction of the middle and distal one third of the proximal phalanx; an attempt should be made to identify and preserve this small cutaneous nerve. The approach exposes the lateral band or intrinsic contribution to the extensor mechanism. Depending on the location of pathology and necessary exposure, the lateral band may be elevated dorsally or a longitudinal split created between the lateral band and the central tendon dorsally. This tendon-splitting approach is more useful when more proximal exposure is required. Distal exposure is easily managed through with elevation or dorsal retraction alone. Burton and Eaton have noted that a triangular portion of the lateral band may be excised to gain additional exposure; however, the authors have not found this technique necessary to achieve sufficient visualization and prefer to preserve the intrinsic contribution to the extensor mechanism.[27] The mid-axial approach may be translated more distally to address condylar fractures of the proximal phalanx as well as fractures at the base of the middle phalanx (see **Fig. 2**B.4). Exposure may be improved by adding a transverse extension across the dorsal PIP extension crease. This is a direct continuation of the incision drawn with the PIP in flexion, continued transversely across the PIP joint.

MIDDLE PHALANGEAL EXPOSURES

Analogous to the proximal phalanx, the middle phalanx may be approached via a dorsal, mid-axial, or volar exposure. The dorsal exposure is useful in repairing or reconstructing central slip injuries and treating fractures, whereas the mid-axial exposure provides excellent exposure for the treatment of fractures and access for the resection of bony tumors. The volar approach is specialized, but affords the greatest access for treating volar base fractures of the proximal phalanx resulting from dorsal PIP dislocation injuries.

The dorsal approach to the middle phalanx is a direct extension of the dorsal approach utilized to access the proximal phalanx (see **Fig. 2**A.7). The incision is placed centrally over the dorsum of the finger. Care should be taken in making the incision, because the central slip of the extensor mechanism inserts onto the underlying middle phalangeal base. The central slip should be preserved in any dorsal exposure to the middle phalanx to avoid creating an iatrogenic boutonniere deformity. The incision may be safely extended proximally across the PIP joint or distally past the DIP joint for sufficient exposure. After identifying the central tendon insertion, the triangular ligament that bridges the lateral bands may be incised or even excised to expose the middle phalangeal diaphysis and condylar region.

The lateral approach to the middle phalanx is a direct extension of the mid-axial approach utilized to access the proximal phalanx (see **Fig. 2**B.3). At this level, one may encounter a dorsal sensory branch arising from the proper digital nerve; however, the branch is often diminutive or absent. Appropriate incision places the proper neurovascular bundles within the volar skin flap. The lateral band is retracted to expose the middle phalanx. Continuation of the incision distal to the DIP places the eponychial branch of the digital nerve at risk and may result in neuroma formation within the contact surface of the finger; consequently, extension distal to the trifurcation is avoided.

The volar approach to the middle phalanx is useful in accessing the PIP joint and the middle phalangeal base (see **Fig. 2**C.2). A Bruner incision is designed over the middle and proximal phalanx. An incision is made and dissection carried directly down to the flexor tendon sheath. The radial and ulnar neurovascular bundles are identified and retracted. The tendon sheath is cleared to define the pulley system. The A-3 pulley lies directly over the PIP joint. The A-2 and A-4 pulleys lie proximal and distal respectively. A window is made between the A-2 and A-4 pulleys, whereas the A-3 pulley is resected or split longitudinally. The FDS and FDP tendons are retracted. It is often easier to retract these tendons in opposing directions to facilitate exposure and a Heiss (cricket) retractor is useful in maintaining this exposure. The A-2 and A-4 pulleys may be partially resected for exposure; however, it is advisable to maintain at least one half of each pulley to prevent postoperative

bowstringing. The volar plate is sharply elevated from the head of the proximal phalanx to see the articular surface of the proximal phalangeal head and distal phalangeal base. The stout volar plate is incised longitudinally on the radial and ulnar aspect, preserving the collateral ligaments as well as a cuff of the proximal edge of the volar plate to allow for subsequent repair with 4-0 Ethibond (Ethicon) sutures. The tendons are allowed to fall back into the fibroosseous tunnel. The authors do not advocate repair of the A-3 pulley because a suture placed in the tendon sheath may create further adhesion; rather, the leaflets of the A-3 pulley are allowed to rest over the tendons. The skin is then closed with interrupted 4-O nylon sutures.[28–30]

DISTAL PHALANGEAL EXPOSURES

The distal phalanx is surgically exposed in a limited number of conditions, namely the treatment of bony mallet injuries with subluxation and the treatment of distal phalangeal nonunions. Bony mallet injuries are exposed from a dorsal approach. A longitudinal incision typically does not provide sufficient distal exposure because the nail plate and germinal matrix limit distal extension. H-Shaped incisions may be designed with the transverse limb centered over the DIP joint (see **Fig. 2**A.5). Mid-axial extensions 0.5 to 0.75 cm in length are designed. Dissection is limited distally to avoid injury to the germinal matrix of the nail complex. The terminal portion of the extensor tendon is typically in continuity with the dorsal bony fragment and this insertion is maintained. The skin is loosely approximated with simple 5-0 nylon sutures to avoid undue tension on the closure.

A volar approach to the distal phalanx allows access to the mid portion and tuft of the distal phalanx, structures that are inaccessible from the dorsal aspect without violating the nail complex. Although the approach places a scar on the volar aspect of the finger tip, central placement within the digital pulp and restriction in distal incision length result in favorable outcomes. The skin is incised sharply, as is the volar pulp. The FDP insertion is preserved and the bone is exposed with a freer elevator. Blunt dissection is avoided because multiple spreads violate the volar pulp structure and result in greater scarring. The skin incision is closed with 4-O nylon sutures.

PEARLS AND PITFALLS

Choosing the appropriate surgical approach to any structure in the hand requires an intricate understanding of the normal anatomy and the pathologic anatomy associated with the particular injury or disease process being treated. In cases of fracture management, the surgeon should have a 3-dimensional picture in mind as to where each of the fracture fragments are located, how they are displaced, and exactly how they will fit together to recreate the alignment of the bone or joint surface. With this mental picture, choosing the most facile approach to achieve a particular end result becomes self-evident.

Incisions should be made sufficiently long for appropriate visualization, intervention (reduction, repair, or excision), and introduction of hardware, if necessary. Lack of appropriate visualization may result in injury to poorly visualized critical structures and a shorter incision will result in a worse scar if the skin edges are traumatized in an effort to attain visualization or in

the introduction of hardware via an undersized exposure.

Consideration should be given to the planned postoperative rehabilitation regimen. For example, a trans-EPL approach to the thumb MCP joint should be avoided if the interphalangeal joint is unstable and cannot be left free in the postoperative splint. A lack of EPL gliding will invariably result in adhesions and stiffness. A volar approach to a middle phalangeal base fracture should not be undertaken if the osseous fixation is not sufficient to tolerate active motion for FDS and FDP tendon gliding.

The functional role of the hand is clear. Because the hand is visible in daily interaction, consideration should be given to its cosmetic appearance. The dorsal surface of the hand is particularly

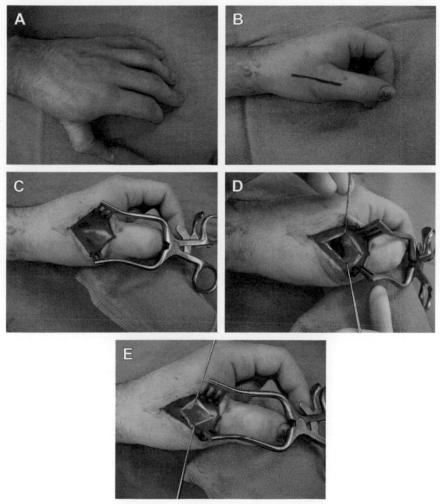

Fig. 5. Trans-EPL approach to the thumb metacarpophalangeal joint. (*A*) Dorsal thumb MCP dislocation. (*B*) Incision placement for trans-EPL approach. (*C*) EPL and EPB tendons exposed. (*D*) EPL tendon divided longitudinally. (*E*) MCP joint post reduction.

prominent from a cosmetic perspective and incisions placed on the dorsal aspect require gentle tissue handling and meticulous surgical closure. When feasible, a midlateral or volar incision that respects the cosmetic and functional units of the hand is preferred. The authors counsel all patients regarding scar management, including scar massage, sun avoidance, and the use of sunscreens and silicone gel sheeting once the wound has healed. Compliance with scar management is often challenging given the mobility of the dorsal hand skin and exposure of the hand in daily activities. These obstacles may be overcome by recommending the use of a liquid or paintable product or use of sheeting at night while the hand is at rest. Incisions placed in midaxial and volar locations are less visible and tend to result in more favorable scars given the lack of tension placed on these repairs with motion of the hand.

ILLUSTRATIVE CLINICAL CASES

Case 1

A 39-year-old, right-hand dominant painter sustained an injury to his left hand. He fell, striking his thumb against a scaffolding cross bar resulting in a dorsal dislocation of the MCP joint. Attempts at closed reduction were unsuccessful and an open reduction was performed through a trans-EPL approach (**Fig. 5**).

Case 2

A 26-year-old man suffered an injury to his left thumb when he fell from a mountain bike. He has laxity to radially directed stress at the MCP joint in full extension and at 30° of flexion. He has a palpable mass on the ulnar aspect of the MCP joint. He underwent open repair of his ulnar collateral ligament injury via a UCL approach (**Fig. 6**).

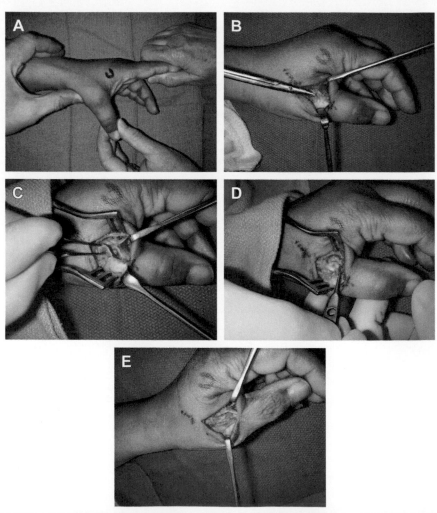

Fig. 6. Thumb UCL repair. (*A*) Laxity of thumb MCP to radially directed stress. (*B*) Ulnar aspect of thumb MCP exposed. Littler scissors indicate the adductor pollicis aponeurosis. Stener lesion. (*C*) Adductor aponeurosis divided. (*D*) UCL with associated radial condylar fragment placed in anatomic position. (*E*) UCL and adductor aponeurosis after repair.

REFERENCES

1. Watt AJ, Friedrich JB, Huang JI. Advance in treating skin defects of the hand: skin substitutes and negative-pressure wound therapy. Hand Clin 2012; 28(4):519–28.
2. Hentz VR, Chase RA. Hand surgery: a clinical atlas. Philadelphia: W.B. Saunders: Harcourt Health Sciences Company; 2001. p. 1–33.
3. Chin SH, Vedder NB. MOC-PS SM CME article: metacarpal fractures. Plast Reconstr Surg 2008; 121(1 Suppl):1–13.
4. Kollitz KM, Hammert WC, Vedder NB, et al. Metacarpal fractures: treatment and complications. Hand (N Y) 2014;9(1):16–23.
5. Woodburne RT, Burkel WE. Essentials of human anatomy. New York: Oxford University Press; 1994. p. 154–69.
6. Lanz U. Anatomical variations of the median nerve in the carpal tunnel. J Hand Surg Am 1977;2(1): 44–53.
7. Burget GC, Menick FJ. The subunit principle in nasal reconstruction. Plast Reconstr Surg 1985; 76(2):239–47.
8. Spear SL, Davison SP. Aesthetic subunits of the breast. Plast Reconstr Surg 2003;112(2):440–7.
9. Hollenbeck ST, Woo S, Komatsu I, et al. Longitudinal outcomes and application of the subunit principle to 165 foot and ankle free tissue transfers. Plast Reconstr Surg 2010;125(3):924–34.
10. Abdel-Rehim S, Kowalski E, Chung KC. Enhancing aesthetic outcomes of soft tissue coverage of the hand. Plast Reconstr Surg, in press.
11. Johnson AE, Bagg MR. Ipsilateral complex dorsal dislocations of the index and long finger. Am J Orthop 2005;34:241–5.
12. Becton JL, Christian JD Jr, Goodwin HN, et al. A simplified technique for treating the complex dislocation of the index metacarpophalangeal joint. J Bone Joint Surg Am 1975;57:698–700.
13. Barry K, McGee H, Curtin J. Complex dislocation of the metacarpophalangeal joint of the index finger: a comparison of surgical approaches. J Hand Surg Br 1988;13:466–8.
14. Bohart PG, Gelberman RH, Vandell RF, et al. Complex dislocations of the metacarpophalangeal joint. Operative reduction by Farabeuf's dorsal incision. Clin Orthop 1982;164:208–10.
15. Adler GA, Light TR. Simultaneous complex dislocation of the metacarpophalangeal joints of the long and index fingers. A case report. J Bone Joint Surg Am 1981;63:1007–9.
16. Mudgal CS, Mudgal S. Volar open reduction of complex metacarpophalangeal dislocation of the index finger. Tech Hand Up Extrem Surg 2006;10(1):31–6.
17. Williams JS Jr, Kamionek S, Weiss AP, et al. The surgical approach in non-border digit complex dislocations of the metacarpophalangeal joint. Orthop Rev 1994;23(7):601–5.
18. Dinh P, Franklin A, Hutchinson B, et al. Metacarpophalangeal joint dislocation. J Am Acad Orthop Surg 2009;17(5):318–24.
19. Kuhn KM, Dao KD, Shin AY. Volar A1 pulley approach for the fixation of avulsion fractures of the base of the proximal phalanx. J Hand Surg Am 2001;26(4):762–71.
20. Hattori Y, Doi K, Sakamoro S, et al. Volar plating for intra-articular fracture of the base of the proximal phalanx. J Hand Surg Am 2007;32(8):1299–303.
21. Kozin SH. Treatment of thumb ulnar collateral ligament ruptures with Mitek bone anchor. Ann Plast Surg 1995;35:1–5.
22. Weiland AJ, Berner SH, Hotchkiss RN, et al. Repair of acute ulnar collateral ligament injuries of the thumb metacarpophalangeal joint with and intraosseous suture anchor. J Hand Surg Am 1997;22:585–91.
23. Stern PJ, Burgess SD, Kubik VD. Open Treatment of Oblique and Spiral Fractures of the Proximal Phalanx. In: Chung KC, editor. Operative techniques: hand and wrist surgery. New York: Elsevier; 2008. p. 28–34.
24. Pun WK, Chow SP, So YC, et al. Unstable phalangeal fractures: treatment by A.O. screw and plate fixation. J Hand Surg Am 1991;16:113–7.
25. Dabezies EJ, Schutte JP. Fixation of metacarpal and phalangeal fractures with miniature plates and screws. J Hand Surg Am 1986;11:283–8.
26. Chamay A. A distally based dorsal and triangular tendinous flap for direct access to the proximal interphalangeal joint. Ann Chir Main 1988;7(2):179–83.
27. Burton RI, Eaton RG. Common hand injuries in the athlete. Orthop Clin North Am 1973;4(3):809–38.
28. Green A, Smith J, Redding M, et al. Acute open reduction and rigid internal fixation of proximal interphalangeal joint fracture dislocation. J Hand Surg Am 1992;17:512–7.
29. Hamilton SC, Stern PJ, Fassler PR, et al. Mini-screw fixation for the treatment of proximal interphalangeal joint fracture dislocations. J Hand Surg Br 2006;31: 1349–54.
30. Lee JY, Teoh LC. Dorsal fracture dislocations of the proximal interphalangeal joint treated by open reduction and interfragmentary screw fixation: indications, approaches and results. J Hand Surg Br 2006;31:138–46.

REFERENCES

Soft Tissue Coverage of the Upper Extremity
An Overview

Harvey Chim, MD[a], Zhi Yang Ng, MRCS[b], Brian T. Carlsen, MD[c],
Anita T. Mohan, MD[c], Michel Saint-Cyr, MD[c],*

KEYWORDS

- Hand • Upper extremity • Soft tissue defect • Soft tissue coverage

KEY POINTS

- Soft tissue defects of the upper extremity require durable coverage that will allow early postoperative mobilization and rehabilitation to maximize functional outcomes.
- Fasciocutaneous flaps are preferable to muscle flaps for coverage of exposed structures, as these result in lesser postoperative adhesions and are easier to elevate secondarily for definitive tendon or nerve reconstruction.
- Early free flap reconstruction may be necessary in cases of high voltage injuries as a procedure for limb salvage, although it must be recognized that flap failure rates are also higher; special consideration for the use of spare parts in cases of unsalvageable amputations is also warranted to reduce further patient morbidity when providing soft tissue cover.
- Various reconstructive modalities are available and described for soft tissue coverage of the upper extremity, but ultimately, treatment should be tailored according to patient-, surgeon-, and defect-specific characteristics.
- The advent of negative pressure wound therapy has obviated the need for emergent wound coverage, and allows stable temporary coverage of the wound prior to definitive reconstruction.

INTRODUCTION

The primary goal of soft tissue coverage in wound management is to allow the underlying defect to heal. In the setting of upper extremity trauma, however, such soft tissue defects are oftentimes compounded in nature because of the involvement of other anatomic structures such as bones, tendons, nerves, vessels, and muscles that are both in close proximity and have important roles in the overall function of the upper limb. Associated defects of these structural components can be addressed by various methods including osteosynthesis, tendinous repairs, nerve coaptations, vascular grafting, and muscle transfers. It is the durable and appropriate soft tissue cover for the wound that is paramount for the proper recovery and rehabilitation of the injured upper extremity.[1]

In preparation for definitive soft tissue coverage of the traumatized upper extremity, there are several basic principles to adhere to. First, early and aggressive debridement of the wound should be performed to remove all contaminated and

The authors have nothing to disclose.
[a] Division of Plastic Surgery, University of Miami Miller School of Medicine, Miami, FL 33136, USA;
[b] Department of Plastic Reconstructive and Aesthetic Surgery, Singapore General Hospital, Outram Road, Singapore 169608, Singapore; [c] Division of Plastic Surgery, Mayo Clinic, 200 First Street Southwest, Rochester, MN 55905, USA
* Corresponding author.
E-mail address: saintcyr.michel@mayo.edu

nonviable tissue. This approach extends from tumor cases in which the wound and its edges are excised in an en bloc fashion.[2] When there are concerns over the adequacy of debridement, such as when tissue viability is equivocal following crush, burn, or electrical injuries, or when the wound is severely contaminated, serial debridement is indicated. This comes at the expense of worsening edema and granulation tissue, however, which may further obscure tissue planes and delay or even impede reconstruction and thus postoperative rehabilitation.[3] Certainly, debridement reduces the risk of wound bed infection, but it is also important in allowing a full assessment of the extent of reconstruction required, because the original defect often becomes much larger than was previously estimated. Stable bone fixation, if necessary, should be attempted next so as to provide a solid framework for the subsequent repair of exposed vital structures.[4] Concerns remain with regard to addressing nerve and tendon defects in the same setting as early definitive soft tissue cover because of the risks of infection and the possibility of consequent nerve or tendon graft loss.[5]

Once the wound bed has been adequately debrided, an osseotendinous framework provided (if necessary), and other involved structures repaired, the reconstructive surgeon is faced with a multitude of considerations in selecting the most appropriate modality to provide definitive soft tissue coverage of the upper extremity (**Fig. 1**). The purpose of this article is to provide an overview of the various options and considerations involved in providing such cover. Specifically, the reconstructive plan should be tailored to address both patient- and defect-specific characteristics such as existing patient comorbidities and the mechanism and extent of injury, respectively.

INDICATIONS/CONTRAINDICATIONS

In general, the reconstructive ladder can be used to approach upper extremity soft tissue defects. Although some wounds may be closed primarily, these are few and far between in trauma. Many defects with no exposed structures, even large ones, may be covered with a split-thickness skin graft. The ideal form of soft tissue reconstruction will

- Allow for the obliteration of dead space to decrease the risk of infection
- Promote wound healing via re-establishment of the venous and lymphatic circulations[6]
- Be vascularized from out of the zone of injury, and particularly in the upper extremity
- Provide a pliable yet robust cover for the smooth gliding and excursion of tendons and muscles such that maximal functional recovery can be achieved (**Fig. 2**).[7]

Although local and regional flaps may be used for coverage of smaller soft tissue defects (**Fig. 3**), larger defects will usually require coverage by free flaps (**Fig. 4**).

By extension, these reconstructive goals should also be achieved as early as possible and ideally, in a 1-stage setting.[8] If free tissue transfer is required, this may be performed emergently, per the landmark work of Godina,[9,10] but equivalent outcomes may be achieved when coverage is

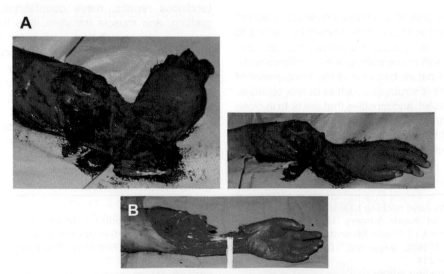

Fig. 1. Predebridement (*A*) and postdebridement (*B*) examples following traumatic injury to left forearm. Early aggressive debridement of the wound should be performed to remove all contaminated and nonviable tissue. This allows for an accurate assessment and planning of reconstructive options.

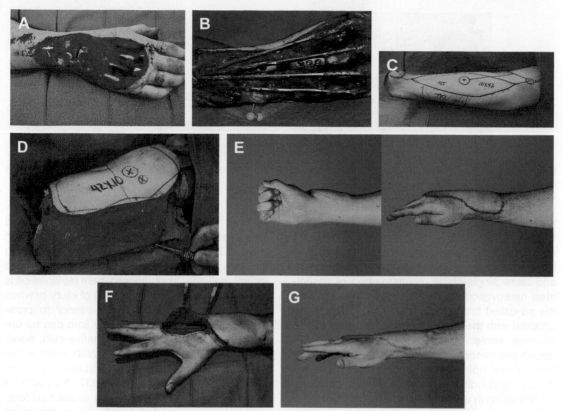

Fig. 2. Right hand dorsal injury with avulsion of soft tissue following roll-over injury crush injury, presenting with soft tissue loss and bony instability. (*A*) Preoperative image following serial debridement. (*B*) Wrist fusion carried out to maintain bony stability and extensor tendon reconstruction with autologous tendon grafts. (*C*) Preoperative marking for planned extended Anterolateral thigh (ALT) fasciocutaneous flap with Fascia Lata extension for soft tissue coverage of plate and tendon grafts, and allow for tendon glide and under the soft tissue reconstruction. (*D*) Extended ALT raised harvested with demonstration of Fascia Lata extension. (*E*) Final result following coverage of ALT flap for wound coverage before secondary flap thinning procedures. (*F*) Extensor lag repair and tenolysis under local anesthesia block and liposuction thinning of ALT flap. (*G*) Final result following secondary procedures.

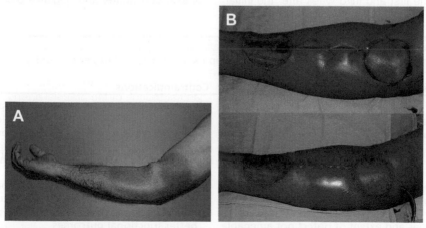

Fig. 3. (*A*) Preoperative clinical photograph of a sarcoma within the antecubital fossa. (*B*) Intraoperative photographs demonstrating suprafascial harvest of a pedicled radial forearm flap for wound coverage and full thickness skin graft from the groin for donor site closure at the wrist.

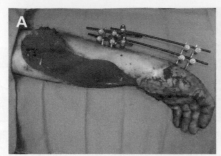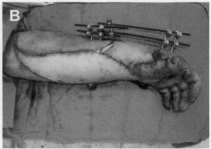

Fig. 4. (*A*) Intraoperative photographs of soft tissue defect on the volar forearm with Ex-fix insitu. (*B*) Soft tissue coverage with free Anterolateral thigh (ALT) flap.

performed within the first week after injury, following adequate serial debridement of the wound, if required. In addition, free flaps can be harvested in a composite or even chimeric fashion and allow single-stage reconstruction of associated neurovascular and osseotendinous defects, the so-called orthoplastic approach.[11] Therefore, coupled with the additional benefits of fewer procedures, earlier postoperative mobilization, and decreased hospital stay and costs overall,[12] it is the authors' opinion that under the right circumstances and indications (**Table 1**) there should be no hesitation in utilizing a free flap.

Special consideration is warranted for burn injuries to the upper extremity (**Fig. 5**) and the concept of the use of spare parts in cases of amputation of the unsalvageable limb. Although early definitive soft tissue coverage is advocated for in the setting of high-impact trauma to reduce the risks of subsequent sepsis, osteomyelitis, and limb loss, free flap coverage in the acute setting for thermal and high voltage burn injuries has been reported to experience higher rates of flap loss and failure, with most incidences occurring within the first and third week after the initial

insult.[13,14] This may be attributed to the masked presentation of the extent of soft tissue destruction in these injuries, but it should also be highlighted that most of these acute free flaps were performed for limb salvage. In situations where replantation is impossible because of the extent of injury or when functional outcomes would be inferior to prosthetic use, the amputated upper limb can be utilized as an excellent donor of native skin, bone, tendons, nerves, vessels, and joints even in the form of spare parts for the reconstruction of composite defects with associated skin loss without further donor site morbidity. The amputated forearm has been reported for its use in the acute setting as a radial forearm free flap to provide both immediate and durable skin cover for padding of the amputation stump and subsequent prosthesis fitting[15,16] while the fillet flap, both pedicled and free, is well described for immediate soft tissue cover using viable components of unsalvageable digits and limbs.[17]

Finally, in cases that are not amenable to early free flap reconstruction, temporary soft tissue cover can still be provided using an ever-increasing array of skin substitutes and negative-pressure wound

Table 1
Indications and contraindications for early free flap reconstruction of upper extremity defects

Indications	Contraindications
Absolute • Exposure of reconstructed, or native and intact vital structures (eg, tendon, bone, joints, vessels) • Exposed hardware Relative • Good functional outcomes are anticipated • Early, aggressive, and adequate debridement can be achieved • Zone of injury precludes the use of local flaps • Dimensions and extent of defect not amenable to simple reconstruction (eg, primary closure, skin grafting)	• Unstable patient or those with multiple co-morbidities who cannot tolerate prolonged anesthesia for complex operative procedures • Heavily contaminated wound requiring serial debridement to achieve a clean wound bed (eg, crush, burn, and blast injuries) • Extensive injury such that radical debridement would render functional restoration unlikely • If amputation and prostheses would provide better functional outcomes • Lack of microvascular expertise and/or facilities

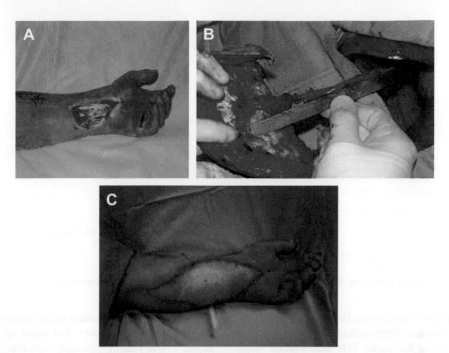

Fig. 5. (*A*) Volar wrist defect following an electrical burn requiring further wound excision and debridement back to healthy tissue, making a much larger defect for soft tissue coverage. (*B, C*) Intraoperative photograph demonstrating the use of an anterolateral thigh (ALT) flap raised with a 15 cm pedicle length to permit vascular anastomosis away from the site of injury and final inset of flap.

therapy. Integra (Integra LifeSciences, Plainsboro, NJ) is a bovine collagen-based scaffold that permits growth of the neodermis and can provide temporary wound coverage prior to definitive split-thickness skin grafting (STSG). Its successful use has been reported for the coverage of exposed tendons, bones, and joints in the hand[18,19] but remains indicated mainly for dorsal hand wounds because of the prolonged period of immobilization necessary for engraftment and take of the neodermis and STSG respectively.[20] Alloderm (Life Cell, Branchburg, NJ), another dermal substitute derived from banked human cadaveric skin, has been reported for acute soft tissue coverage in deep hand burns with exposed underlying structures in patients not suitable for immediate flap coverage.[21] Cadaveric skin allografts can be used as a biological dressing for temporary wound coverage of exposed vital structures prior to definitive skin grafting.

The advent of negative pressure wound therapy (VAC dressings) has resulted in a paradigm shift in soft tissue coverage, obviating the need for emergent free tissue transfer for coverage of exposed structures. In cases in which the patient is not fit for surgery because of other injuries or in which the wound bed is not ready, VAC dressings reduce edema and keep the wound clean, allowing for dressing changes to be performed at longer intervals. VAC dressings also serve to bolster and promote skin graft take and skin substitute incorporation[22,23] for coverage of soft tissue defects of the upper extremity.

ALGORITHM FOR THE SELECTION OF TYPE OF SOFT TISSUE COVERAGE

Various reconstructive algorithms[7] have been proposed, but ultimately, it is a cogent and individualized approach toward addressing all relevant aspects of upper extremity soft tissue defects that is vital for a successful outcome. The authors propose an algorithm (**Fig. 6**) for upper extremity soft tissue cover based on patient- and defect-specific characteristics (**Table 2**) while adhering to the reconstructive principles of adequate wound bed preparation, respecting the zone of injury, and replacing like with like.

Muscle-only and myocutaneous flaps such as the latissimus dorsi (LD) and rectus abdominis have traditionally been used for dead space obliteration due to their bulky nature and for combating wound bed infection through enhanced blood supply and thus antibiotic delivery. However, the postoperative adhesions associated with these muscle flaps may render delayed

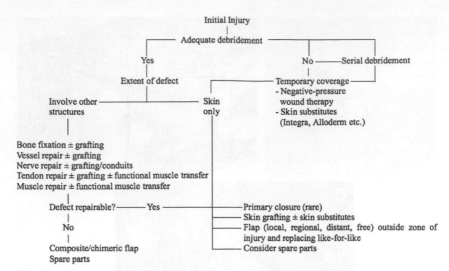

Fig. 6. Proposed reconstructive algorithm for soft tissue coverage of the upper extremity.

reconstruction of underlying tendinous, nerve, and other structural defects difficult during secondary flap elevation. As such, fasciocutaneous flaps have gained increasing popularity due to easier elevation in a delayed setting. Moreover, these flaps are able to provide a better match for the color and contour of the defect due to a greater range of donor site choices (such as the anterolateral thigh [ALT] flap, lateral arm flap, radial forearm flap, deep inferior epigastric perforator [DIEP] flap) and may be harvested as perforator flaps to further decrease flap bulk and donor site morbidity.[5] By extension, fasciocutaneous flaps can be modified and harvested as even thinner fascial flaps (**Fig. 7**). This is particularly advantageous for the coverage of exposed tendons to prevent further desiccation while allowing smooth tendon glide to prevent the build-up of adhesions.[24] The main drawback, however, would be the need for skin grafting over the fascia for definitive wound closure and thus a second donor site. When compound defects of the upper extremity occur, various composite flaps incorporating different components can be utilized such as the osteocutaneous fibula free flap for segmental bone loss. Chimeric flaps, in which different tissue types and portions based on their individual vascular supply that merge into 1 parent pedicle, have found increasing application as demonstrated by the use of various components of the subscapular system for complex upper limb reconstruction.[25]

Table 2
Patient- and defect-specific characteristics to be considered prior to definitive coverage for upper extremity soft-tissue defects

Considerations	Implications
Patient-Specific • Current medical condition and existing co-morbidities (eg, ischemic heart disease, diabetes mellitus) • Hand dominance, profession • Habitus	• Unstable patients or those with multiple co-morbidities may not be able to tolerate prolonged, complex microsurgical procedures • Functional vs complete reconstruction • Bulk of a particular flap may vary between patients (eg, anterolateral thigh) and affect flap choicea
Defect-Specific • Mechanism of injury • Extent of injury • Location and dimensions of injury	• Crush, blast and burn injuries may require serial debridement and temporary coverage • If direct repair of damaged structures cannot be achieved, composite or chimeric flaps may be required • Deliberation between fasciocutaneous, fascial, myocutaneous, and muscle-only flaps whilst balancing the need to replace "like with like"

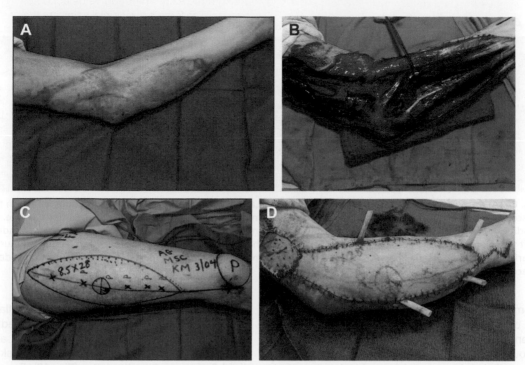

Fig. 7. (A) Preoperative image of a patient with a ulna nerve palsy secondary to a neuroma, strongly positive at the elbow, and an unstable skin graft which was predisposed to breakdown. (B) Intraoperative image following excision of skin graft and excision of neuroma followed by sural nerve cable grafting. (C) An ALT flap from the right thigh was planned following Doppler assessment, to provide good color match, contour and adequate padding and support. (D) Intraoperative image following inset.

The use of negative-pressure wound therapy and various forms of skin substitutes for temporary soft tissue coverage has been expounded upon previously. The various techniques of osteosynthesis, tendinous repair and grafting, vascular anastomosis including the use of interposition vein grafts, neurorrhaphy, and nerve grafts or conduits are all well described in the literature and beyond the scope of this article. Here the focus will be on the various flap options for upper extremity defects, specifically of the upper arm and shoulder, forearm and elbow, and hand and fingers. The authors also advocate an approach to flap choice by local and distant (free) options, and in the case of the former, consideration of potential flap options both proximal and distal to the zone of injury.

Upper Arm and Shoulder

Soft tissue defects of the upper arm and shoulder are less common compared with of the forearm and hand. However, trauma affecting this region and the resultant soft tissue defect can lead to contour irregularities with possible extension to involve exposure of the glenohumeral and acromioclavicular joints, as well as peripheral neurovascular structures. Flaps vascularized from outside the zone of injury would include those based on the different branches of the subclavian system proximally (latissimus dorsi [LD] and trapezius flaps) as well as free flaps. The LD muscle supplied by the thoracodorsal artery[26] and its variations[27] are commonly employed both as a pedicled or free muscle-only or myocutaneous flap and have consistently achieved successful results in terms of wound healing, minimal donor site morbidity, and good functional outcomes (**Figs. 8** and **9**); the serratus can also be harvested at the same time for additional bulk if required. Other recently described options include the fasciocutaneous lateral arm flap, which can be rotated up to 180° or advanced proximally on its pedicle to provide coverage for defects up to 5 × 15 cm² in size.[28] The fasciocutaneous trapezius flap which can be designed based on its lower muscle fibers to avoid glenohumeral disruption, which can occur in LD flap harvest, has a long arc of rotation to reach up to the shoulder tip,[29] or utilized in the setting of distal subclavian artery thrombosis following trauma.[30] These flaps can also be designed to incorporate vascularized bone segments

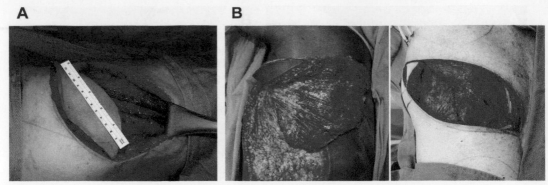

Fig. 8. (*A*) Intraoperative photograph of muscle sparing Latissimus dorsi flap with the skin paddle, based on the descending branch of the thoracodorsal artery and demonstrating the splitting of the latissimus dorsi muscle. (*B*) Traditional latissimus dorsi muscle harvest which results in a greater degree of undermining of the surrounding soft tissue and increased dead space (*Left*). Comparison showing the donor site bed following a pedicled muscle sparing latissimus dorsi flap harvest, which required minimal undermining under skin flaps and reduction in dead space.

from the humerus (lateral arm), rib, or scapula (LD) as osteocutaneous flaps as required. Finally, as mentioned previously, the use of spare parts should always be considered, especially in cases where limb salvage is not amenable; Lee reported a fillet of upper arm pedicled flap based on the brachial artery and provided immediate soft tissue cover of 25 × 15 cm[231] albeit in a tumor case, but its applicability in the setting of trauma is evident.

Forearm and Elbow

Soft tissue coverage for forearm defects become increasingly complicated as the neurovascular and tendinous structures are closer to the subcutaneous layer. Soft tissue defects of the elbow also present a particular reconstructive challenge because of the constant exposure to external shear and stress. The choice of flap cover in these injuries depends largely on the extent of associated defects.

Local and regional flap options in these cases are usually limited because of their proximity to the zone of injury. However, the proximally based radial forearm fasciocutaneous flap remains a viable option for defects involving the proximal forearm, including the region of the antecubital fossa (see **Fig. 3**), due to a long pedicle (based on the radial artery) of up to 20 cm. The skin cover thus provided is thin and pliable to provide an excellent gliding surface for the underlying tendons. A preoperative Allen test is mandatory, however, prior to radial artery sacrifice and a major drawback is the need for skin grafting of the donor site, although there have been reports of modifications to flap harvest such that a pure fascial flap can be harvested to allow primary closure of the

donor site.[32] The pedicled lateral arm and LD flaps as previously described can also be extended to reach distally and provide cover for elbow and proximal forearm defects albeit at a higher risk of distal flap necrosis in the latter (**Fig. 10**). For defects located over the distal forearm, the radial forearm flap can be based distally and harvested in a reversed fashion. Zancolli also described the posterior interosseous flap based on the posterior interosseous artery[33] to circumvent the donor site morbidities associated with the radial forearm flap, and the reach of the posterior interosseous flap can extend beyond distal forearm defects to reach up to the metacarpal joints and the first web space.

Free flap reconstruction of forearm defects affords the greatest versatility, however, due to the option of incorporating various soft tissue components in a compound or chimeric fashion. For resurfacing of shallow defects of the upper extremity, the anterolateral thigh (ALT) flap is currently the method of choice, because it

- Is of moderate thickness
- Has a long pedicle (descending branch of the lateral circumflex femoral artery) to allow revascularization well beyond the zone of injury
- Provides a large area of cutaneous coverage of up to 30 cm in length
- Has a donor site that can be closed primarily[10]

Especially for volar forearm defects with tendon exposure, the ALT can be thinned primarily[34] or harvested as a fascia-only flap. The ALT can also be harvested to incorporate the fascia lata, the lateral femoral cutaneous nerve, and even part of the iliac crest for tendon reconstruction, restoration

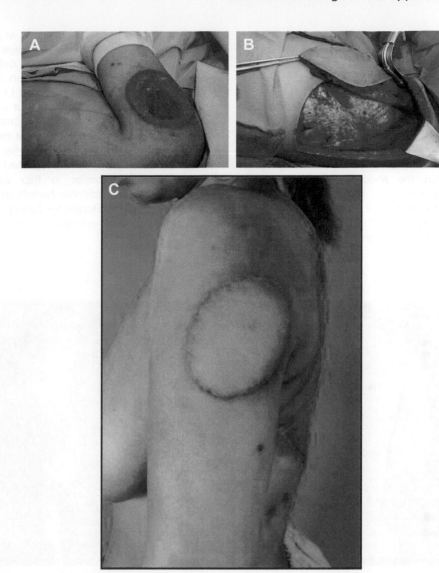

Fig. 9. (*A*) Intraoperative image following sarcoma excision postero-lateral left arm. (*B*) Pedicled Latissimus Dorsi muscle raised. (*C*) Final postoperative clinical photograph.

of protective sensation, and primary bone grafting, respectively.[35] Similar reconstructive outcomes can be achieved with the thoracodorsal artery perforator (TAP) flap and other fasciocutaneous flaps based on the subscapular system. These flaps can also be expanded as required by incorporating part of the LD or serratus muscles[36] to cover larger defects, or include a segment of scapula for composite reconstruction; sensory restoration, however, is not usually attainable. For resurfacing of deeper and more complex defects, the bulk associated with the LD or rectus abdominis may be more suitable.[37] The free rectus abdominis is usually harvested based on the deep inferior epigastric artery and can provide an area of

coverage of up to 21 × 14 cm². [38] Sensation can also be provided through the inclusion and neurorraphy of an intercostal nerve. The morbidity associated with a free rectus abdominis flap in the form of abdominal wall weakness and hernias can be avoided by a muscle-sparing harvest, or raising of the flap based on the deep (DIEP) or superficial inferior epigastric arteries (SIEA); its main advantage over the LD and ALT flaps is the obviated need for a change in patient position intraoperatively. When reconstructive requirements are more extensive, such as in soft tissue defects with segmental bone loss, various options are available depending on the length of bone required. Most commonly, the osteocutaneous fibula free flap is harvested with a vascularized bone segment (up to 25 cm in length[39]) based on the peroneal artery, and a cuff of soleus can also be included for dead space obliteration. Other options include the iliac crest as part of the deep circumflex iliac artery (DCIA) flap, scapula as part of the LD/TAP flap, distal radius as part of the radial forearm flap, and a segment of the humerus as part of the lateral arm flap.

In terms of elbow coverage, various local and distant flaps have been described. Although local flaps including the anconeus, brachioradialis, flexor carpi ulnaris, and triceps have all been described with successful outcomes, these usually lie within the zone of injury in the setting of upper extremity trauma and hence, may be less than optimal for soft tissue coverage. In addition, these local flaps only allow for coverage of small defects. The workhorse flap for large defects still remains the radial forearm flap. Caution, however, is raised for the use of the pedicled LD flap for elbow defects extending beyond the olecranon due to the risk of distal flap necrosis from increased stretch and tension on the muscle; in such cases, either the pedicled radial forearm flap or free tissue transfer is advocated to avoid the potential compromise in flap vascularity (see **Fig. 10**).[40] An additional benefit to the use of the LD flap is the potential for functional restoration of flexion and extension of the elbow if needed.[41]

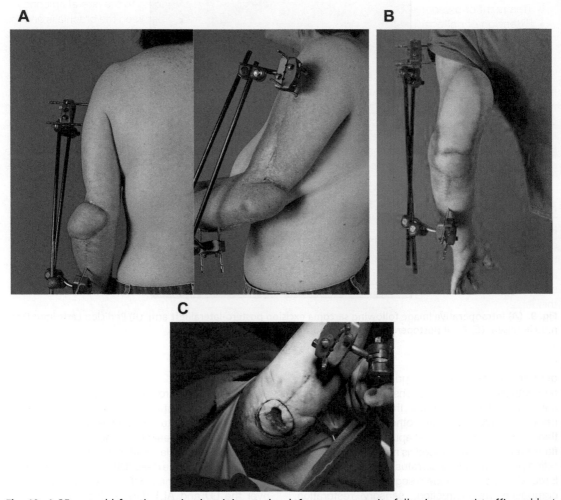

Fig. 10. A 35 year old female sustained an injury to her left upper extremity following a road traffic accident, referred following a pre-expanded pedicled lateral arm flap for soft tissue reconstruction and with a spanning external fixator in-situ and significant contour deformity. (*A*) Preoperative clinical images demonstrating significant contour deformity at the elbow. (*B*) Initial postoperative photograph following pedicled LD reconstruction and re-positioning of the lateral arm flap toward the original donor site. (*C*) Subsequent wound break down at the distal edge of LD flap. (*D*) Following debridement, a pedicled suprafascial radial forearm flap was used to cover the defect at the elbow, with a full thickness skin graft from the groin for the donor site wound.

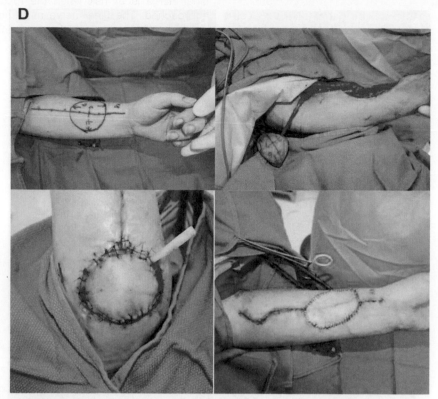

D

Fig. 10. (*continued*)

Hand and Fingers

Hand and finger soft tissue defects are the most common due to their role in everyday living. It is this functional role, however, that gives rise to anatomic differences between the dorsal and volar surfaces of the hand. Dorsal skin of the hand is thinner and looser to enable tendon excursion, while volar skin is thicker and tougher while still allowing motion and tactile sensation through a glaborous surface. Therefore, donor site selection in soft tissue reconstruction of the hand and finger defects is usually the hand itself because of optimal and specialized tissue match for superior functional and sensory restoration. Distant options would require a balance between the functional outcomes that can be achieved with additional donor site morbidity and less than optimal cosmesis.

When used on other parts of the upper extremity, STSGs are usually meshed to provide coverage of larger defects. Meshing of skin grafts for soft tissue coverage of the injured hand is avoided,[7] however, due to the increased risk of contractures, especially over the web spaces and crease folds. Therefore, in consideration of the properties of hand skin, unmeshed STSGs and full-thickness skin grafts (FTSGs) are commonly used for dorsal (and larger)

and volar (and smaller) defects, respectively. The skin harvested for FTSGs should also be glabrous in nature, and commonly used donor sites include hairless areas such as the ipsilateral hypothenar eminence, medial plantar arch, volar wrist, and groin crease.

For dorsal skin defects of the hand, local reconstructive options include the reversed radial forearm flap and the posterior interosseous artery flap as described previously, and the Becker flap based on the dorsal ulnar artery,[42] which can provide an area of coverage of up to 20 × 9 cm^2.[43] With more extensive defects, free flaps can be designed in various configurations such as muscle-only, fascial, and fasciocutaneous as required, and common donor sites include the lateral arm (**Fig. 11**), ALT, LD, and rectus abdominis. When the LD or rectus is chosen, modified harvest of only the superior portion of the LD or a partial medial rectus flap can be performed for less donor site morbidity and decreased bulk for better contour matching.[44] For extensive defects with extensor tendon exposure, the temporoparietal fascial flap based on the superficial temporal artery can provide well-vascularized tissue for skin graft take and is also durable enough for

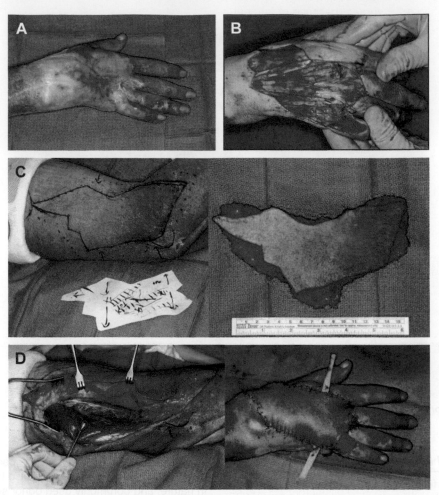

Fig. 11. (*A*) Burn wound contracture on dorsum of right hand causing limitations in finger flexion and hand function. (*B*) Post burn wound excision. (*C*) Custom lateral arm flap designed from wound template following burn wound excision and harvested as free fasciocutaneous flap. (*D*) Intraoperative identification of perforators from the posterior collateral artery and final inset to dorsum of hand.

mechanical stability to allow early rehabilitation, although it is limited in size to about 14 × 12 cm^2.[45] For even larger defects, the serratus fascia flap can be harvested for coverage of up to 15 × 20 cm^2 and may also be extended in chimeric fashion to include components of the subscapular system for more complex reconstruction. When local and free flap reconstructions are not possible, the use of skin substitutes such as Integra with STSG remains a viable option. Similarly, local pedicled options for volar defects of the hand can be provided using the reversed radial forearm flap, dorsal ulnar artery flap, and posterior interosseous artery flap. Free flap options include those as described before, and increasingly, there is a greater appreciation of the gracilis flap due to its suitable size, consistent anatomy of the vascular pedicle based on the medial circumflex

femoral artery system, minimal donor site morbidity, and the ability to be transplanted as a free-functioning muscle transfer (FFMT) for associated loss of musculature[46,47] and function. Novel free flap options recently described for simultaneous FFMT reconstruction of thenar defects include the use of gracilis[47] and ipsilateral anconeus.[48] Finally, the use of spare parts is argued for when indicated and a fillet of a finger flap with its constituent bones and tendons removed can be used for coverage of defects adjacent to the unsalvageable digit.

Isolated soft tissue defects of the fingers and fingertips are usually addressed with local flap coverage and may require additional skin grafts. For distal fingertip defects with exposure of the distal phalanx, the V-Y advancement flap and its various modifications (bilateral, oblique) have been described to provide both soft tissue cover and sensation[49] by incorporating the digital neurovascular bundles. When more than a third of the volar tissue of the fingertip is lost, the cross-finger flap and its variations (Hueston, Souquet, Turkish)[49–51] and the thenar flap (for index and long fingers only) are among the many options available. In situations in which the donor flap cannot merely be advanced, they can be designed in an island fashion pedicled on the digital neurovascular bundle to reach greater distances. These are known as homo- or heterodigital island flaps, and commonly described options include

- Homodigital island advancement flap (can be designed in anterograde or retrograde[52,53] fashion) for the fingers
- Moberg thumb advancement flap[54] for thumb defects of the distal phalanx
- Dorsal metacarpal artery flap[55] for thumb and dorsal hand defects
- Littler flap[56] for thumb defects

Because the skin of the fingers does not have much tissue laxity, most of these flaps will require skin grafting of the donor site.

COMPLICATIONS AND MANAGEMENT

Following the provision of soft tissue cover, various potential complications and consequent sequelae may still occur. Skin grafts and skin substitutes may fail to engraft should the wound bed be inadequately prepared or infection occurs, and they may also be sheared off if not protected properly. Later-onset complications may include contractures, especially if sited over web spaces and joint creases, thereby causing restricted tendon motion; hypopigmentation leading to a less than ideal aesthetic result, especially over exposed surfaces of the upper extremity such as the forearm and hand dorsum, and affect cosmesis if harvested from a nonhairless area. Flap complications can be broadly classified as acute or late. Early signs of venous congestion may be addressed with simple maneuvers such as loosening overlying dressings, but if not improving, these signs may necessitate a return to the operating room for the exploration of the venous anastomosis. Similarly, clinical signs of arterial thrombosis will also necessitate operative re-exploration and may require refashioning of the anastomosis; if areas of demarcation start to present, operative debridement is obligated to salvage the flap. Other possible complications of later onset may include wound dehiscence and flap or fat necrosis, which again may also ultimately culminate with flap loss.

Other soft tissue-related complications include those affecting the associated structures of the skin, bones and joints, tendons and muscles, and nerves such as scar contractures, osteomyelitis, joint stiffness and arthrosis, scarring and adhesions, fibrosis and disuse atrophy, neuromas, and complex regional pain syndrome, respectively. These can be addressed by various secondary procedures such as scar revisions, capsulotomies, tenolysis, and sympathectomies that are beyond the scope of this article.

POSTOPERATIVE CARE

Free flap reconstruction requires routine postoperative monitoring as per individual institution practices, and valuable adjuncts may include implantable Doppler probes. The key toward optimizing functional outcomes in the traumatized upper extremity with reconstructed soft tissue defects is early and aggressive mobilization once the construct is deemed viable and the surrounding edema has subsided. Prior to that, volar hand injuries with flexor tendon involvement and that of the dorsum with repaired extensor tendons are managed with dynamic splinting[57] and assisted active range of motion exercises, respectively.

OUTCOMES

A recent systematic review concluded that there was no significant difference in flap-related complications with regard to the timing of post-traumatic upper extremity microsurgical reconstruction.[58] It is argued that the original recommendations by Godina for early free flap reconstruction within 72 hours, which was later reaffirmed by Ninkovic[59] and Lister,[8] may no longer be absolute because of the increasingly recognized and successful role of negative-pressure wound therapy as a temporizing measure before second-look debridements for clearer demarcation of non-viable tissue and, in accordance with the principles of adequate debridement and anastomosis outside the zone of injury, better preparation of the wound bed prior to definitive reconstruction.[60,61] The corollary to this is that early reconstruction would be easier to perform, because overall, there would be less edema, inflammation, propensity for vessel thrombosis, and likelihood for infection, but the operating surgeon must ensure that adequate wound debridement had been carried out.

SUMMARY

Under the right conditions, early microsurgical reconstruction of soft tissue defects of the traumatized upper extremity can lead to favorable outcomes and enable the patient to return to a high level of function. When the patient is not fit to undergo early free flap transfer, other options available include local and regional flaps and temporary soft tissue coverage using a variety of skin substitutes and negative-pressure wound therapy. The, former, however, may be harvested within close proximity to the zone of injury and is thus associated with the attendant increased risk of vascular thrombosis and flap failure, while the latter may allow for equivocal wounds to be debrided adequately prior to definitive wound coverage. Increasing knowledge of vascular supply and flap anatomy will lead to more innovative flaps being designed with the potential for compound and/or chimeric applications in this challenging and important area of reconstructive surgery.

REFERENCES

1. Eberlin KR, Chang J, Curtin CM, et al. Soft-tissue coverage of the hand: a case-based approach. Plast Reconstr Surg 2014;133(1):91–101.
2. Scheker LR, Ahmed O. Radical debridement, free flap coverage, and immediate reconstruction of the upper extremity. Hand Clin 2007;23(1):23–6.
3. Sundine M, Scheker LR. A comparison of immediate and staged reconstruction of the dorsum of the hand. J Hand Surg Br 1996;21(2):216–21.
4. Brenner P, Lassner F, Becker M, et al. Timing of free microsurgical tissue transfer for the acute phase of hand injuries. Scand J Plast Reconstr Surg Hand Surg 1997;31(2):165–70.
5. Neumeister M, Hegge T, Amalfi A, et al. The reconstruction of the mutilated hand. Semin Plast Surg 2010;24(1):77–102.
6. Slavin SA, Upton J, Kaplan WD, et al. An investigation of lymphatic function following free-tissue transfer. Plast Reconstr Surg 1997;99(3):730–43.
7. Giessler GA, Erdmann D, Germann G. Soft tissue coverage in devastating hand injuries. Hand Clin 2003;19(1):63–71.
8. Lister G, Scheker L. Emergency free flaps to the upper extremity. J Hand Surg Am 1988;13(1):22–8.
9. Godina M. Early microsurgical reconstruction of complex trauma of the extremities. Plast Reconstr Surg 1986;78(3):285–92.
10. Saint-Cyr M, Gupta A. Indications and selection of free flaps for soft tissue coverage of the upper extremity. Hand Clin 2007;23(1):37–48.
11. Levin LS. The reconstructive ladder. An orthoplastic approach. Orthop Clin North Am 1993;24(3):393–409.
12. Derderian CA, Olivier WA, Baux G, et al. Microvascular free-tissue transfer for traumatic defects of the upper extremity: a 25-year experience. J Reconstr Microsurg 2003;19(7):455–62.
13. Baumeister S, Köller M, Dragu A, et al. Principles of microvascular reconstruction in burn and electrical burn injuries. Burns 2005;31(1):92–8.
14. Sauerbier M, Ofer N, Germann G, et al. Microvascular reconstruction in burn and electrical burn injuries of the severely traumatized upper extremity. Plast Reconstr Surg 2007;119(2):605–15.
15. Rees MJ, de Geus JJ. Immediate amputation stump coverage with forearm free flaps from the same limb. J Hand Surg Am 1988;13(2):287–92.
16. Brown RE, Wu TY. Use of "spare parts" in mutilated upper extremity injuries. Hand Clin 2003;19(1):73–87.
17. Küntscher MV, Erdmann D, Homann HH, et al. The concept of fillet flaps: classification, indications, and analysis of their clinical value. Plast Reconstr Surg 2001;108(4):885–96.
18. Weigert R, Choughri H, Casoli V. Management of severe hand wounds with Integra® dermal regeneration template. J Hand Surg Eur Vol 2011;36(3):185–93.
19. Taras JS, Sapienza A, Roach JB, et al. Acellular dermal regeneration template for soft tissue reconstruction of the digits. J Hand Surg Am 2010;35(3):415–21.
20. Watt AJ, Friedrich JB, Huang JI. Advances in treating skin defects of the hand: skin substitutes and negative-pressure wound therapy. Hand Clin 2012;28(4):519–28.
21. Bhavsar D, Tenenhaus M. The use of acellular dermal matrix for coverage of exposed joint and extensor mechanism in thermally injured patients with few options. Eplasty 2008;8:e33.
22. Blackburn JH 2nd, Boemi L, Hall WW, et al. Negative-pressure dressings as a bolster for skin grafts. Ann Plast Surg 1998;40(5):453–7.
23. Kim EK, Hong JP. Efficacy of negative pressure therapy to enhance take of 1-stage allodermis and a split-thickness graft. Ann Plast Surg 2007;58(5):536–40.
24. Flügel A, Kehrer A, Heitmann C, et al. Coverage of soft-tissue defects of the hand with free fascial flaps. Microsurgery 2005;25(1):47–53.
25. Boa O, Servant JM, Revol M, et al. Dorsal decubitus positioning: a novel method to harvest the latissimus dorsi flap for massive upper extremity defect reconstruction. Tech Hand Up Extrem Surg 2011;15(3):166–71.
26. Ma CH, Tu YK, Wu CH, et al. Reconstruction of upper extremity large soft-tissue defects using pedicled latissimus dorsi muscle flaps—technique illustration and clinical outcomes. Injury 2008;39(Suppl 4):67–74.
27. Wong C, Saint-Cyr M. The pedicled descending branch muscle-sparing latissimus dorsi flap for trunk and upper extremity reconstruction. J Plast Reconstr Aesthet Surg 2010;63(4):623–32.

28. Jordan SW, Wayne JD, Dumanian GA. The pedicled lateral arm flap for oncologic reconstruction near the shoulder. Ann Plast Surg 2013. http://dx.doi.org/10.1097/SAP.0b013e3182853f0b.

29. Rasheed MZ, Tan BK, Tan KC. The extended lower trapezius flap for the reconstruction of shoulder tip defects. Ann Plast Surg 2009;63(2):184–7.

30. Satish C. Reconstruction of complex shoulder defect in a case of subclavian artery thrombosis. Indian J Surg 2013;75(Suppl 1):366–7.

31. Lee GK, Mohan SV. Complex reconstruction of a massive shoulder and chest wall defect: de-bone appétit flap. J Surg Case Rep 2010;3:1.

32. Reyes FA, Burkhalter WE. The fascial radial flap. J Hand Surg Am 1988;13(3):432–7.

33. Zancolli EA, Angrigiani C. Posterior interosseous island forearm flap. J Hand Surg Br 1988;13(2):130–5.

34. Chen HC, Tang YB. Anterolateral thigh flap: an ideal soft tissue flap. Clin Plast Surg 2003;30(3):383–401.

35. Meky M, Safoury Y. Composite anterolateral thigh perforator flaps in the management of complex hand injuries. J Hand Surg Eur Vol 2013;38(4):366–70.

36. Izadi D, Paget JT, Haj-Basheer M, et al. Fasciocutaneous flaps of the subscapular artery axis to reconstruct large extremity defects. J Plast Reconstr Aesthet Surg 2012;65(10):1357–62.

37. Horch RE, Stark GB. The rectus abdominis free flap as an emergency procedure in extensive upper extremity soft-tissue defects. Plast Reconstr Surg 1999;103(5):1421–7.

38. Mathes SJ, Nahai F. Reconstructive surgery: principles, anatomy & technique. New York: Churchill Livingstone; 1997.

39. Berger RA, Weiss AP. Hand surgery. Philadelphia: Lippincott Williams & Wilkins; 2004.

40. Choudry UH, Moran SL, Li S, et al. Soft-tissue coverage of the elbow: an outcome analysis and reconstructive algorithm. Plast Reconstr Surg 2007;119(6):1852–7.

41. Brones MF, Wheeler ES, Lesavoy MA. Restoration of elbow flexion and arm contour with the latissimus dorsi myocutaneous flap. Plast Reconstr Surg 1982;69(2):329–32.

42. Becker C, Gilbert A. Le lambeau cubital. [The cubital flap]. Ann Chir Main 1988;7:136–42 [in French].

43. Holevich-Madjarova B, Paneva-Holevich E, Topkarov V. Island flap supplied by the dorsal branch of the ulnar artery. Plast Reconstr Surg 1991;87(3):562–6.

44. Parrett BM, Bou-Merhi JS, Buntic RF, et al. Refining outcomes in dorsal hand coverage: consideration

of aesthetics and donor-site morbidity. Plast Reconstr Surg 2010;126(5):1630–8.

45. Upton J, Rogers C, Durham-Smith G, et al. Clinical applications of free temporoparietal flaps in hand reconstruction. J Hand Surg Am 1986;11(4):475–83.

46. Krimmer H, Hahn P, Lanz U. Free gracilis muscle transplantation for hand reconstruction. Clin Orthop Relat Res 1995;(314):13–8.

47. Baker PA, Watson SB. Functional gracilis flap in thenar reconstruction. J Plast Reconstr Aesthet Surg 2007;60(7):828–34.

48. Ng ZY, Lee SW, Mitchell JH, et al. Functional anconeus free flap for thenar reconstruction: a cadaveric study. Hand (N Y) 2012;7(3):286–92.

49. Chao JD, Huang JM, Wiedrich TA. Local hand flaps. J Am Soc Surg Hand 2002;1(1):25–44.

50. Cronin T. The cross finger flap: a new method of repair. Am Surg 1951;17:419–25.

51. Atasoy E. Reversed cross-finger subcutaneous flap. J Hand Surg Am 1982;7A:481–3.

52. Lai CS, Lin SD, Yang CC. The reverse digital artery flap for fingertip reconstruction. Ann Plast Surg 1989;22(6):495–500.

53. Kojima T, Tsuchida Y, Hirasé Y, et al. Reverse vascular pedicle digital island flap. Br J Plast Surg 1990;43(3):290–5.

54. Moberg E. Aspects of sensation in reconstructive surgery of the upper extremity. J Bone Joint Surg Am 1964;46:817–25.

55. Holevich J. A new method of restoring sensibility to the thumb. J Bone Joint Surg Br 1963;45:496–502.

56. Littler JW. Neurovascular pedicle transfer of tissue in reconstructive surgery of the hand. J Bone Joint Surg Am 1956;38:917–23.

57. Scheker LR, Langley SJ, Martin DL, et al. Primary extensor tendon reconstruction in dorsal hand defects requiring free flaps. J Hand Surg Br 1993;18(5):568–75.

58. Harrison BL, Lakhiani C, Lee MR, et al. Timing of traumatic upper extremity free flap reconstruction: a systematic review and progress report. Plast Reconstr Surg 2013;132(3):591–6.

59. Ninkovic M, Deetjen H, Ohler K, et al. Emergency free tissue transfer for severe upper extremity injuries. J Hand Surg Br 1995;20(1):53–8.

60. Kumar AR, Grewal NS, Chung TL, et al. Lessons from the modern battlefield: successful upper extremity injury reconstruction in the subacute period. J Trauma 2009;67(4):752–7.

61. Steiert AE, Gohritz A, Schreiber TC, et al. Delayed flap coverage of open extremity fractures after previous vacuum-assisted closure (VAC) therapy: worse or worth? J Plast Reconstr Aesthet Surg 2009;62(5):675–83.

Soft Tissue Coverage of the Arm

Paul Binhammer, MSc, MD, FRCS(C)

KEYWORDS

- Soft tissue • Arm • Latissimus dorsi • Flap

KEY POINTS

- The latissimus dorsi is supplied by the thoracodorsal artery, which divides into the transverse and descending branch allowing the muscle to be split. There is a secondary supply from intercostal perforators.
- A skin paddle is usually taken based on perforators from descending branches along the anterior border of the muscle.
- Using the latissimus dorsi as a functional muscle requires placing the muscle on stretch, marking with sutures, and then replicating this at the time of reinsertion.
- The donor site may develop a seroma and the use of drains is advised.

INTRODUCTION

The arm presents with fewer challenges for soft tissue coverage than the rest of the upper extremity. The arm tends to be less exposed to trauma than the hand. The muscles about the arm are larger than those of the forearm, providing greater coverage for the humerus. Excluding the elbow and shoulder, the anterior aspect of the arm is covered by the biceps and brachialis, whereas the posterior aspect is covered by the triceps. Median and ulnar nerves along with the brachial artery are medial, whereas the radial nerve passes from proximal to distal by way of the spiral groove.

Although there are nerve and vascular structures, there are not the flexor and extensor tendons that require coverage, as found in the forearm and even more so in the hand. Thus in many situations coverage can be achieved by skin grafting. In addition, the greater circumference of the arm provides more available tissue from which to gain primary closure of local random pattern flaps.

The presence of the latissimus dorsi muscle in close proximity, its relative ease of dissection, and the ability to tailor it for large or small defects has meant that it serves as the main muscle for

arm coverage.[1–7] Although there is a case report of using an expanded scapular flap, the latissimus dorsi is the flap of choice.[8]

LATISSIMUS DORSI

The use of the latissimus dorsi as a musculocutaneous pedicled flap is more than 100 years old.[9] It is large and thin, allowing it to cover substantial defects and mold into cavities. It can be raised with overlying skin or can be part of a chimeric flap using the subscapular system.[10]

The vascular pattern of the muscle is type 5, having a dominant blood supply from the thoracodorsal artery and a secondary supply of perforators from the intercostals. Within the muscle, the thoracodorsal divides into a descending branch and a transverse branch 94% of the time.[11] The motor nerve supply is the thoracodorsal nerve, which divides into 2 branches following the descending and transverse arterial branches. The muscle inserts into the medial lip of the bicipital groove, after twisting 180°, and arises from the lower 6 thoracic vertebrae and to the iliac crest by way of the thoracolumbar fascia. Other points of origin include the tip of the scapula, the lower

The author has nothing to disclose.

Division of Plastic Surgery, University of Toronto, 2075 Bayview Avenue, Toronto, Ontario M4N 3M5, Canada

E-mail address: p.binhammer@utoronto.ca

Hand Clin 30 (2014) 475–478

http://dx.doi.org/10.1016/j.hcl.2014.07.005

4 ribs, and portions of serratus. The function of the muscle is to push off or draw the humerus down to the side from a flexed posture as in cross-country skiing. Along with the teres major, it forms the posterior axillary fold.

The anatomy of the latissimus dorsi allows coverage of substantial areas, although the proportion farthest away from the pedicle posterior and inferior may not survive.[12] It can be tailored as a partial muscle flap by taking the anterior border with only the descending branch. The vascular pedicle can be isolated and the nerve preserved to the portion that is left intact.

Skin can be taken with the muscle and a paddle is generally reliable anywhere along the midportion of the muscle. However, there are a significant number of cutaneous perforators 2 to 4 cm posterior to the anterior border, which enhance reliability and flexibility of the flap.[13,14] Although incorporating a skin flap has advantages in particular situations it increases the bulk of the flap and this should be taken into consideration. A skin graft helps to decrease bulk. When an innervated muscle is not required, denervation of the muscle allows for atrophy, which may improve contour in some situations.

Because the vascular pedicle is long and the insertion is on the humerus, the muscle covers both the arm and elbow at the same time.[15] There is a large amount of undermining because of the broad flat muscle, so postoperative seroma can occur. The use of suction-assisted drains for a prolonged period of time (2 weeks or more) is advised. Harvesting can be done endoscopically.[16]

The muscle has also been used both for coverage and simultaneously for elbow or shoulder function (most commonly elbow flexion[3–5,7,17]). It is important to mark the tension of the muscle with sutures before detachment. When subsequently performing appropriate proximal and distal fixation, the correct tension must be set based on the distance between the sutures. Postoperative splinting and therapy are keys for success.

OPERATIVE TECHNIQUE

The defect to be covered and the length of muscle required based on the anatomy of the insertion point are planned before surgery, along with whether and where a skin paddle needs to be placed. The steps of the operation, depending on the complexity, are visualized and written out.

The anterior margin of the muscle can be marked by asking the patient to adduct against resistance. If the patient is unable to do so, the anterior margin of the muscle can be estimated by drawing from the posterior axillary fold to the midline of the iliac crest. The muscle will be slightly posterior to this estimate. The superior margin of the muscle can be drawn in a curving line from the point of insertion to the thoracic spine, passing just superior to the inferior angle of the scapula.

A skin pedicle can be marked out with its long axis paralleling that of the anterior border of the muscle and beginning below the posterior axillary fold. The central axis of the skin paddle should be over the perforators, approximately 4 cm posterior to the muscle margin. A template of the defect can be used to design the skin flap, although a flap of 10 cm in width is approximately the size that can be easily closed.

The patient is prepped and draped in the lateral decubitus position with the arm free, draped, and resting on a Mayo stand. The arm can be moved throughout the procedure to avoid any position that may stretch the brachial plexus.

The anterior incision is made in the skin flap, or, when not using a skin paddle, the skin is incised along the anterior margin of the muscle. The muscle margin is identified and any adjustment of skin markings can be performed.

Lift the skin of the back off the muscle for the desired length of muscle based on preoperative planning. Elevate the muscle off the chest wall beginning at least 12 cm away from the humerus and working away from the vascular pedicle, which protects the pedicle. Slips to serratus and the lower ribs have to be divided. Intercostal perforators need to be clipped.

At this point, the surgeon should be able to see the deep and superficial planes of the muscle with attachments inferior, along the spine and scapula. The area about the neuromuscular pedicle has not been dissected. Divide the muscle distally accounting for some extra because of contracture, and reflect the muscle toward the humerus to continue the deep dissection of the pedicle.

Depending on how much rotation and mobility are required, the surgeon can now dissect the vascular pedicle and nerve, and divide the point of insertion. Vascular branches to the serratus anterior and the chest wall may have to be divided.

THORACODORSAL ARTERY PERFORATOR FLAP

The thoracodorsal artery perforator flap uses the perforators from the descending branch that pass through the latissimus dorsi muscle into the skin.[13,14] The skin for this flap overlies the anterior border of the muscle. Although this does not provide as large an area of tissue for coverage, it does spare the muscle. Its marking and elevation are similar to those of the latissimus dorsi flap,

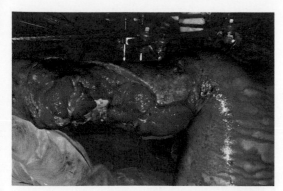

Fig. 1. Posterior view of arm defect 3 weeks after improvised explosive device.

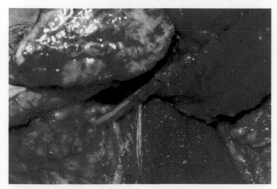

Fig. 2. Split latissimus dorsi with skin paddle.

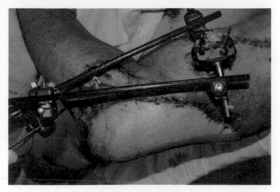

Fig. 3. Preserved transverse branch nerve.

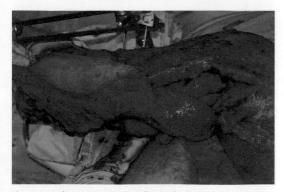

Fig. 4. Early postoperative lateral view.

as indicated earlier; however, the flap is raised as a perforator flap.[18]

Figs. 1–4 show cases representing the topics discussed in this article.

REFERENCES

1. Germann G, Steinau HU. Functional soft-tissue coverage in skeletonizing injuries of the upper extremity using the ipsilateral latissimus dorsi myocutaneous flap. Plast Reconstr Surg 1995;96(5):1130–5.
2. Sadove RC, Vasconez HC, Arthur KR, et al. Immediate closure of traumatic upper arm and forearm injuries with the latissimus dorsi island myocutaneous pedicle flap. Plast Reconstr Surg 1991;88(1): 115–20.
3. Rogachefsky RA, Aly A, Brearley W. Latissimus dorsi pedicled flap for upper extremity soft tissue reconstruction. Orthopedics 2002;25(4):403.
4. Stevenson TR, Duus EC, Greene TL, et al. Traumatic upper arm defects treated with latissimus dorsi muscle transposition. J Pediatr Orthop 1984;4(1):111.
5. Minami A, Ogino T, Ohnishi N, et al. The latissimus dorsi musculocutaneous flap for extremity reconstruction in orthopedic surgery. Clin Orthop 1990; 260:201.
6. Behnam AB, Chen CM, Pusic AL, et al. The pedicled latissimus dorsi flap for shoulder reconstruction after sarcoma resection. Ann Surg Oncol 2007;14(5):1591–5.
7. Stern PJ, Carey JP. The latissimus dorsi flap for reconstruction of the brachium and shoulder. J Bone Joint Surg Am 1988;70(4):526–35.
8. Russell RC, Khouri RK, Upton J, et al. The expanded scapular flap. Plast Reconstr Surg 1995; 96(4):884–95 [discussion: 896–7].
9. Tanzini I. Sepra il mio nuovo processo di amputazione della mammella. Reforma Med 1906;12:757.
10. Bakhach J, Peres JM, Scalise A, et al. The quadrifoliate flap: a combination of scapular, parascapular, latissimus dorsi and scapula bone flaps. Br J Plast Surg 1996;49(7):477–81.
11. Bartlett SP, May JW Jr, Yaremchuk MJ. The latissimus dorsi muscle: a fresh cadaver study of the primary neurovascular pedicle. Plast Reconstr Surg 1981;67(5):631–6.
12. Manktelow RT. Latissimus dorsi in microvascular reconstruction anatomy applications and surgical technique. Berlin: Springer-Verlag; 1986. p. 45.
13. Schaverien M, Wong C, Bailey S, et al. Thoracodorsal artery perforator flap and latissimus dorsi myocutaneous flap–anatomical study of the constant skin paddle perforator locations. J Plast Reconstr Aesthet Surg 2010;63(12):2123–7.
14. Thomas BP, Geddes CR, Tang M, et al. The vascular basis of the thoracodorsal artery perforator flap. Plast Reconstr Surg 2005;116:818.

15. Chang LD, Goldberg NH, Change B, et al. Elbow defect coverage with a one-staged, tunneled latissimus dorsi transposition flap. Ann Plast Surg 1994; 32(5):496.

16. Lin CH, Wei FC, Levin LS, et al. Donor-site morbidity comparison between endoscopically assisted and traditional harvest of free latissimus dorsi muscle flap. Plast Reconstr Surg 1999;104(4):1070–7.

17. Pierce TD, Tomaino MM. Use of the pedicled latissimus muscle flap for upper-extremity reconstruction. J Am Acad Orthop Surg 2000;8(5):324–31.

18. Koshima I, Narushima M, Mihara M, et al. New thoracodorsal artery perforator (TAPcp) flap with capillary perforators for reconstruction of upper limb. J Plast Reconstr Aesthet Surg 2010;63(1): 140–5.

Soft Tissue Coverage of the Elbow

Amitava Gupta, MD, FRCS[a],*, Zach Yenna, MD[b]

KEYWORDS

- Pedicled flaps • Free flaps • Elbow defects • Elbow coverage

KEY POINTS

- Small defects of the posterior elbow can be covered with local flaps.
- Moderate defects require regional pedicled flaps. We prefer the antegrade posterior interosseous artery flap for posterior elbow coverage.
- Large defects of the elbow will require space-filling muscle free flaps. Half of the latissimus dorsi or gracilis are the free flaps that we favor.

INTRODUCTION

Soft tissue defects about the elbow may arise from a variety of insults to the upper extremity, including blunt and penetrating trauma, burns, infection, tumor resection, or from sequelae of prior treatment and associated patient morbidity.

These defects expose a complex set of anatomic structures that must be attended to, including bone, vessels, nerves, ligaments, muscles, tendons, and possibly implants, all while minimizing the functional and cosmetic deficits imposed by the reconstructive process.

Options available for soft tissue coverage are dependent on the patient's age, overall health, size of the soft tissue defect and associated injuries, availability of tissue, and socioeconomic factors, including expectations, work and family demands, and ability to care for the wound in the postoperative period.

Soft tissue coverage begins with primary closure of a wound and advances to increasingly more complex and demanding solutions, free tissue transfers, in what has been described as the reconstructive ladder.[1] The correct solution is the simplest one that minimizes patient morbidity, provides for a predictable return to function, and takes into consideration the previously mentioned patient factors.

Our discussion considers pedicled flaps about the elbow and free flaps. Local pedicle flaps are indicated in situations in which anatomic structures or implants are exposed and are absent native tissue or blood supply, or are at risk of infection.

Absolute contraindications to these flaps are few and include damage to the flap's vascular supply, those flaps that would compromise distal blood supply to the extremity, and possibly those patients with musculocutaneous, median, or radial nerve deficits where the flap may otherwise be used to restore function about the elbow.

Relative contraindications are varied, and include the patient's age, nutritional status, and associated comorbidities, such as diabetes, peripheral vascular disease, or tobacco use.

RADIAL FOREARM FLAP

The radial forearm flap (RFF) was performed in the 1970s by Chinese surgeons and was described to the West in 1982 by Song and colleagues.[2] The RFF is a fasciocutaneous flap that offers reliable and versatile coverage of elbow wounds, incorporating thin, pliable tissue. It can also meet the demands of incorporating sensate soft tissue coverage as well as vascularized bone graft.

The authors have nothing to disclose.
[a] Louisville Arm & Hand, Louisville, KY 40202, USA; [b] Department of Orthopedic Surgery, University of Louisville, Louisville, KY 40202, USA
* Corresponding author.
E-mail address: armhand@gmail.com

hand.theclinics.com

The foundation of the RFF is the proximal aspect of the radial artery, just beyond its emergence from the brachial artery. The distal limit of the RFF is the wrist flexion crease, and it is designed to include up to the volar two-thirds of the forearm. Because of this, the flap may have a long vascular leash and this affords a rotational zone for soft tissue coverage that can span the medial, lateral, dorsal, or volar aspects of the elbow.

If sensation is required, the lateral antebrachial cutaneous nerve of the forearm may be lifted with the cephalic vein to provide a neurotized fasciocutaneous flap. If vascularized bone graft is required for proximal ulna or radial bone defects, or for distal humeral bone defects, the anterolateral aspect of the distal radius can be incorporated.

Downsides to this flap include sacrificing the radial artery as well as donor site morbidity and cosmesis. The flap should be avoided in those patients with a compromised ulnar artery or an incomplete palmar arch. I feel that it is too much to sacrifice such a major artery for carrying a small amount of skin. Moreover, more elegant alternatives exist for elbow coverage.

LATERAL ARM FLAP

The lateral arm flap (LAF) was described separately by Song and colleagues[3] and Katsaros and colleagues[4] for the coverage of head and neck wounds in a free-flap technique. This flap is based proximally on the posterior radial collateral artery. Muruyama and Takeuchi[5] described a modification of this as a rotational flap using the radial recurrent and posterior interosseous recurrent arteries. In this setting, this flap can be used to cover soft tissue defects at the elbow in similar fashion to the RFF.

The LAF can cover defects at any aspect of the elbow, although its rotational zone and overall area of coverage are smaller than that of the RFF. The LAF can incorporate vascularized bone from the humerus and can accommodate the need for sensate coverage with incorporation of the posterior brachial cutaneous nerve.

Advantages of this flap choice include the potential for less donor site morbidity, earlier return to motion at the elbow, and preservation of major arterial blood supplies to the distal extremity.

Disadvantages include the potential for sensory deficits in the zone of the posterior brachial cutaneous nerve, as well as an unsightly scar at the lateral aspect of the arm.

PEDICLE MUSCLE FLAPS FOR SMALL WOUNDS OF THE ELBOW

A variety of flap options exist for coverage of the elbow based on nearby muscular structures, including the flexor carpi ulnaris flap, the brachioradialis flap, and the anconeus muscle flap. Although some of these may be designed to contain overlying cutaneous tissue, it is frequently such that a split-thickness skin graft will be required for superficial coverage of the wound and possibly aspects of the donor site.

The flexor carpi ulnaris (FCU) flap is available to reliably cover anterior elbow soft tissue defects. Proximally, the muscle has 2 origins, that of the medial epicondyle of the humerus and of the proximal ulna, whereas distally the FCU blends into the connective tissue investing the pisiform. The vascular supply of the FCU arises from the posterior ulnar recurrent artery, whereas the nervous supply is derived from perforating branches of the ulnar nerve just distal to the media epicondyle.

The FCU flap has a number of advantages: it is the superficial-most muscle of the volar-ulnar forearm and as such dissection is straightforward. Subsequently, the flap can be accessed rapidly. The flap is primarily indicated for defects of the antecubital fossa, although investigators have described successful approaches to contain posterior defects of the elbow as well.[6]

The brachioradialis (BR) flap is based on the most superficial muscle belly of the mobile wad of the forearm. Although this unit is an important flexor of the elbow, if other flexors are intact, this flap can be performed with minimal functional loss of the extremity.

The muscle arises proximally from the lateral supracondylar ridge of the humerus, between the triceps and brachialis muscles, whereas distally it inserts onto the radial styloid. The vascular supply of the BR flap may arise from the brachial artery, the radial artery, or most commonly the radial recurrent artery. Owing to the length of the muscle, the potential range of rotation for the BR flap is very good. Rohrich and Ingram[7] reported in a cadaveric study that 100% of anterior elbow wounds up to 3 cm in size could be covered by the BR flap, whereas 91% of posterior elbow wounds up to 3 cm could be covered.

The anconeus muscle (AM) flap has been described for posterior wound coverage of the elbow up to 7 cm. Although small, it is immediately accessible at the posterior elbow for coverage of wounds overlying the olecranon, distal triceps, or radiocapitellar joint.

The muscle originates along the lateral epicondyle of the humerus and inserts onto the olecranon. The vascular supply of the muscle is from a variety of sources, although the most important vessel on which to base the flap is the medial collateral artery.

Although the range of the AM flap is limited owing to its size, it is viewed as an expendable muscle that demonstrates little or no morbidity for the patient. Elhassan and colleagues[8] reported on a series of patients with chronic posterior elbow wounds for which the AM flap was used and found no complications, and all had improved range of motion and function of the elbow 1 year postoperatively.

PEDICLE MUSCLE FLAP FOR MODERATE AND LARGE WOUNDS OF THE ELBOW

The most readily available and useful muscle flap for coverage of large defects of the elbow and arm is the latissimus dorsi pedicled flap. This flap has been covered in detail elsewhere within this issue in Paul Buinhammer's article, "Soft Tissue Coverage of the Arm" and will not be discussed here. The latissimus dorsi pedicled muscle flap is great for coverage of posterior arm defects especially when we require a motor substitute for the triceps at the same time. However, generally I have found that it barely reaches the elbow and often the tip of the flap that is the most vital part dies exposing the joint (**Figs. 1** and **2**). Also, I feel that there is great tissue wastage if one uses it to cover an elbow defect.

POSTERIOR INTEROSSEOUS ARTERY FLAP

One of the most versatile soft tissue flaps available for elbow coverage that is reliable, quick, and easy to perform, with minimal donor defect and without the sacrifice of a major blood vessel is the antegrade posterior interosseous artery (PIN) flap. Moreover, a large amount of vascularized fascia can be dissected with the flap and it can be useful in lining the elbow joint or any exposed implant and provides good solution for synovial fistulas.

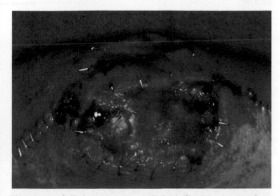

Fig. 1. A full latissimus pedicled flap was used to cover a large posterior elbow defect. The tip of the flap covering the most vital defect became necrotic. (*Courtesy of* A. Gupta, MD, Louisville, KY.)

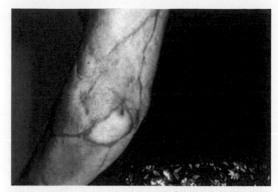

Fig. 2. Salvage of the internal fixation of the elbow with a PIN flap. (*Courtesy of* A. Gupta, MD, Louisville, KY.)

The retrograde posterior interosseous artery flap has been well described in the literature.[9,10] It is a fasciocutaneus flap supplied by perforators from the posterior interosseous artery.

The posterior interosseous artery arises from the interosseous trunk that is a branch of the ulnar artery. In 10% of cases, the posterior interosseous artery arises directly from the ulnar artery. In the proximal forearm, the artery and the accompanying venae commitantes are in intimate and contact with the posterior interosseous nerve with the motor branch to the extensor carpi ulnaris crossing over the vessels on its way to the muscle.

The artery with the venae commitantes then lie between the extensor carpi ulnaris muscle and the extensor digit minimi and run in that plane to just proximal to the wrist. Proximal to the distal radioulnar joint, it gives a radiocarpal branch, a branch to the ulnar head, and the main artery anastomoses with the anterior interosseous artery. During its course in the forearm, it gives 9 to 14 perforators that supply most of the dorsal skin of the forearm.

The procedure for raising an antegrade posterior interosseous artery flap is somewhat different from that of a retrograde posterior interosseous artery flap used for coverage of hand defects. First, the perforators are outlined with a Doppler and marked on the skin. The skin paddle is positioned distally in the forearm so that it can be rotated to cover the elbow. The point of rotation is proximal at the origin of the posterior interosseous artery from the interosseous trunk. The distance from this point to the proximal extent of the elbow defect is measured and imposed distally on the path of the pedicle on the forearm between the fifth and the sixth extensor compartments. The skin paddle is marked distally along this line. The donor defect can be primarily closed when it is up to 3 cm wide. Beyond that, skin grafting will be necessary. First the skin paddle is raised with some extra fascia. Proximal to the proximal extent of the skin paddle, the fascia over the extensor digiti minimi (EDM) and the extensor carpi ulnaris (ECU) are divided longitudinally, preserving the strip of fascia between the two. The posterior interosseous artery pedicle resides in this strip of fascia. Now the distal part of the pedicle is clipped and the skin paddle along with the pedicle is dissected proximally. It is important to be very careful with the dissection as we proceed proximally, as the terminal branches of the posterior interosseous nerve come in close contact with the pedicle. One has to dissect the pedicle carefully away from these branches, taking care not to skeletonize the pedicle. On reaching the origin of the posterior interosseous artery from the posterior interosseous trunk, the flap is now ready to be rotated proximally to cover the defect.

The redundant fascia can be nicely tucked into the depths of the defect and sutured in place with nonabsorbable sutures. Mostly, skin-to-skin apposition of the flap to the donor area is possible. However, if the closure appears too tight, a small skin graft may be applied over the pedicle.

Generally, this flap has been very reliable. There may be some venous congestion that quickly resolves with elevation of the limb.

Case 1

This 43-year-old patient had a severe postburn contracture (**Figs. 3–5**). There were some skin grafts on the posterior aspect of the elbow that broke down after the contracture was released and the patient developed a synovial fistula. A 7 × 3-cm PIN flap was used with a generous amount of forearm fascia to line the joint and provide soft tissue coverage resulting in good functional outcome and complete wound healing.

Case 2

After complex reconstruction of an elbow fracture, the posterior skin defect developed exposing the

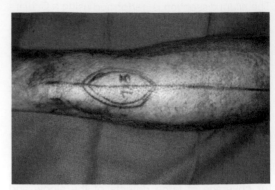

Fig. 4. A 7 × 3-cm posterior interosseous artery flap is planned distally in the forearm centered between the fifth and sixth dorsal compartments. (*Courtesy of* A. Gupta, MD, Louisville, KY.)

olecranon screw (**Fig. 6**). Successful coverage was provided by an antegrade PIN flap.

Case 3

A long and skinny defect over the posterior aspect of the elbow needed coverage after removal of infected total elbow implants (**Figs. 7** and **8**). The patient's elbow was immobilized with an external fixator. A long PIN flap was harvested in an antegrade fashion and the pedicle was tunneled under the skin to reach the recipient site.

Case 4

This young man had the "Ten Commandments" tattooed on the posterior aspect of his forearm (**Figs. 9** and **10**). To cover an indolent nonhealing wound after excision of an olecranon bursa, 3 of the commandments had to be moved with the PIN flap to cover the posterior aspect of his elbow!

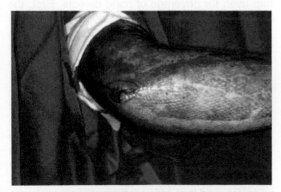

Fig. 3. A synovial fistula developed after release of post burn contracture of the elbow. (*Courtesy of* A. Gupta, MD, Louisville, KY.)

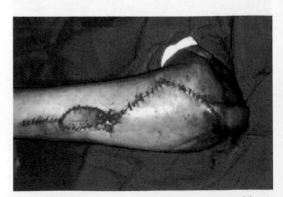

Fig. 5. The skin paddle and generous amount of fascia is used to cover the synovial fistula. (*Courtesy of* A. Gupta, MD, Louisville, KY.)

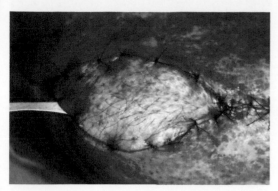

Fig. 6. Coverage of exposed hardware at the tip of the olecranon with a moderate-sized PIN flap. (*Courtesy of* A. Gupta, MD, Louisville, KY.)

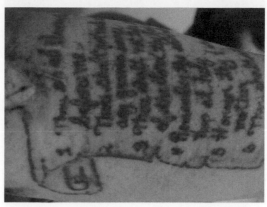

Fig. 9. This patient had the "Ten Commandments" tattooed on the back of his forearm. (*Courtesy of* A. Gupta, MD, Louisville, KY.)

FREE FLAPS

In rare instances, when there is a very large defect of the elbow and distal arm, local soft tissue is not sufficient to cover these defects. Rather than pulling a latissimus dorsi pedicle flap, we believe it is better to plan well and use an appropriate-sized muscle flap with some skin over it as a free flap to cover such a defect. The flaps that are used for such an endeavor include the latissimus dorsi free flap, the rectus abdominis free flap, or the gracilis muscle free flap. The whole or a part of the latissimus dorsi muscle may be harvested. These free flaps have been discussed exhaustively elsewhere.

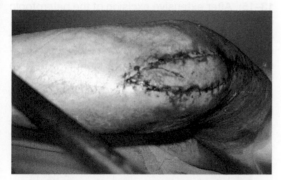

Fig. 7. Coverage of a long posterior defect with a PIN flap. (*Courtesy of* A. Gupta, MD, Louisville, KY.)

Case 5

This 12-year-old boy had a large malignant soft tissue tumor excised from the posterior aspect of the elbow (**Figs. 11** and **12**). The resultant large defect

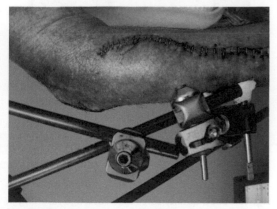

Fig. 8. The pedicle was tunneled under the skin to reach the recipient site. (*Courtesy of* A. Gupta, MD, Louisville, KY.)

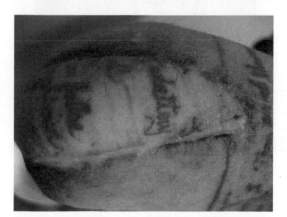

Fig. 10. Three of the commandments were moved to cover his nonhealing wound over the posterior elbow. (*Courtesy of* A. Gupta, MD, Louisville, KY.)

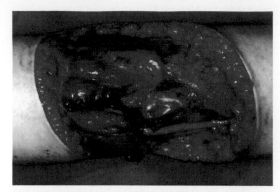

Fig. 11. Large elbow defect after tumor excision in a child. (*Courtesy of* A. Gupta, MD, Louisville, KY.)

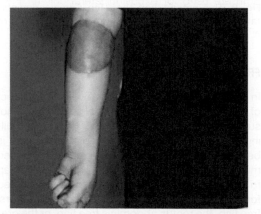

Fig. 12. Coverage of the defect with half latissimus dorsi free flap. (*Courtesy of* A. Gupta, MD, Louisville, KY.)

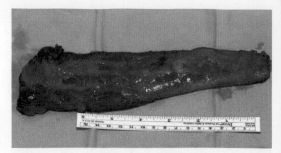

Fig. 14. The gracilis muscle is harvested as a free flap. (*Courtesy of* A. Gupta, MD, Louisville, KY.)

was covered with half latissimus dorsi free flap with skin graft over the muscle. This resulted in good coverage with minimum donor morbidity.

Case 6

This man developed massive heterotopic ossification around his right elbow after head injury (**Figs. 13–15**). After extensive excision of the heterotopic ossification, the posterior wound broke down, exposing the whole elbow joint. The resultant large defect was debrided and covered with a free gracilis flap with skin graft over the flap. We were able to continue mobilizing the patient's elbow, resulting in a good aesthetic and functional result with minimum donor morbidity.

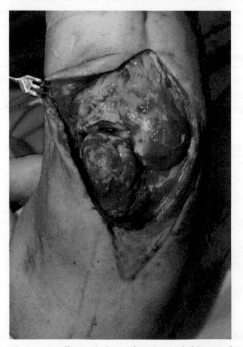

Fig. 13. Large elbow defect after loss of skin resulting from excision of heterotopic bone from the elbow. (*Courtesy of* A. Gupta, MD, Louisville, KY.)

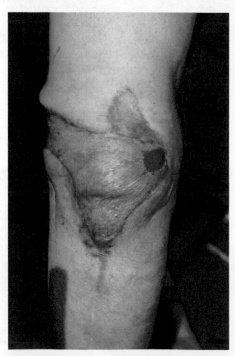

Fig. 15. Good-quality soft tissue coverage resulting in good functional and aesthetic result with minimum donor morbidity. (*Courtesy of* A. Gupta, MD, Louisville, KY.)

REFERENCES

1. Gottleib LJ, Krieger LM. From the reconstructive ladder to the reconstructive elevator. Plast Reconstr Surg 1994;93:1503–4.
2. Song R, Gao Y, Song Y, et al. The forearm flap. Clin Plast Surg 1982;9:21–6.
3. Song R, Song Y, Yu Y, et al. The upper arm free flap. Clin Plast Surg 1982;9:27–35.
4. Katsaros J, Schusterman M, Beppu M, et al. The lateral upper arm flap: anatomy and clinical applications. Ann Plast Surg 1984;12:489–500.
5. Muruyama Y, Takeuchi S. The radial recurrent fasciocutaneous flap: reverse upper arm flap. Br J Plast Surg 1986;39:458–61.
6. Roukoz S. Musculocutaneous flexor carpi ulnaris flap for reconstruction of posterior cutaneotricipital defects of the elbow. Plast Reconstr Surg 2003;111:330–5.
7. Rohrich RJ, Ingram AE. Brachioradialis muscle flap: clinical anatomy and use in the soft-tissue reconstruction of the elbow. Ann Plast Surg 1995;35:70–6.
8. Elhassan B, Karabekmez F, Hsu CC, et al. Outcome of local anconeus flap transfer to cover soft tissue defects over the posterior aspect of the elbow. J Shoulder Elbow Surg 2011;20:807–12.
9. Zancolli EA, Angrigiani C. Posterior interosseous island forearm flap. J Hand Surg Br 1988;13:130–5.
10. Penteado CV, Masquelet AC, Chevrel JP. The anatomic basis of the fascio-cutaneous flap of the posterior interosseous artery. Surg Radiol Anat 1986;8(4):209–15.

REFERENCES

Hand Flaps

Harvey Chim, MD[a], Zhi Yang Ng, MRCS[b], Brian T. Carlsen, MD[c],
Anita T. Mohan, MD[c], Michel Saint-Cyr, MD[c],*

KEYWORDS

- Hand • Upper extremity • Flap • Reconstruction • Soft tissue • Review

KEY POINTS

- The hand is often subject to trauma of various causes which can lead to a variety of injuries to the soft tissue envelope with concomitant involvement of the fingertips, nailbed, and underlying osseotendinous and neurovascular structures.
- The complex structural makeup and functional requirements of the hand necessitate careful consideration of the particular case presented when flap coverage is required.
- Many reconstructive options are available, including local and distally based flaps, and the onus is on the surgeon to carefully weigh up the pros and cons of each technique to address the specific requirements of each individual case.
- The determination of a flap's success is the extent of functional restoration of the patient's injured hand whilst not neglecting potential sequelae, such as suboptimal cosmesis and the lack of cortical reorganization.

INTRODUCTION

By virtue of its predominant role as a tool for communicating with the external environment, the hand is uniquely adapted both in structure and function. Yet, it is also this functional purpose that subjects the unsuspecting hand to myriad injuries, especially trauma, which can occur in the form of crush, blast, degloving, amputation, and burn injuries, among others, and lead to compromise of the soft tissue envelope with resulting functional impairment of the hand.

The reconstructive ladder is well established for wound coverage in general but an ever-increasing number of flap options have been described to address the specific functional and anatomic requirements in soft tissue reconstruction of the hand. First, the loss of mobility in the injured hand contributes to the build-up of edema, scar and tendinous adhesions, and joint contractures. Therefore the necessity to maintain movement is

in direct conflict with the obligated, short period of immobilization required after surgery to allow sufficient wound healing prior to early and active rehabilitation. Second, in comparison with other parts of the body where there is generally adequate skin, fat, and muscle for primary or secondary wound closure, the associated vital structures of the hand are usually located just beneath the enveloping soft tissue layer,[1] and because they are also usually avascular in nature, the use of simpler, lower-rung reconstructive techniques, such as skin grafting, becomes limited. Finally, anatomic differences in different parts of the hand necessitate different considerations—the fingertips are highly specialized structures with a high density of pacinian corpuscles for discriminatory pressure sensation; the dorsal surface has thin, loose, and mobile skin to allow smooth tendon glide whereas the palmar skin is glabrous in nature to withstand the constant external forces associated with working with the hands and

The authors have nothing to disclose.
[a] Division of Plastic Surgery, University of Miami Miller School of Medicine, Miami, FL 33136, USA;
[b] Department of Plastic Reconstructive and Aesthetic Surgery, Singapore General Hospital, Outram Road, Singapore 169608, Singapore; [c] Division of Plastic Surgery, Mayo Clinic, 200 First Street Southwest, Rochester, MN 55905, USA
* Corresponding author.
E-mail address: saintcyr.michel@mayo.edu

hand.theclinics.com

contribute to prehensile function through the formation of skin creases and folds. Therefore, local tissue is often the reconstructive method of choice because it provides optimal tissue match and limits donor site morbidity to the same area to avoid the immobilization of other joints. It is limited in mobility and availability, however, hence usually indicated for smaller sized defects only. With larger hand wounds, regional or free tissue transfer is usually required but this comes at the expense of additional donor site morbidity and suboptimal cosmesis that must be justified to seek a balance with the anticipated functional outcomes.[2]

As with all traumatic wounds, adequate débridement to prepare the wound bed is an absolute maxim prior to flap coverage for definitive wound closure. The choice of flap cover then depends on a thorough assessment of the location, size, and extent of the defect.

INDICATIONS/CONTRAINDICATIONS

The principles of soft tissue reconstruction of the hand have been well described by Beasley[3]: (1) the restoration of sensation with durable cover for normal functional use, (2) minimal donor site morbidity, and (3) the use of reliable techniques with consistent results. Often, hand injuries are not amenable to primary closure, and healing by secondary intention is rarely indicated due to mobility requirements. The use of spare parts should also always be considered when conventional flap reconstruction cannot be achieved.

Defects of the Thumb and Fingertips

Small fingertip defects without exposure of the distal phalanx can usually be left to heal either by secondary intention with epithelialization from the wound edges or covered with a full- or split-thickness skin graft taken from the hypothenar eminence or the volar surface of the forearm. When there is exposure of the underlying bone, flap coverage is indicated (**Table 1**) and may be performed more easily after bone shortening (**Fig. 1**), although this is not without its limitations (discussed later). In larger defects with further exposure of the joint or tendons, more tissue is required and homodigital neurovascular island flaps are usually indicated because they may be advanced further, include the digital nerve for sensory restoration, or even incorporate vascularized tendon (**Figs. 2** and **3**).[4] Compared with the thenar and cross-finger flaps (and its variations), homodigital neurovascular island flaps avoid the need for prolonged immobilization due to the necessity for secondary division, thus reducing the risk of joint stiffness. For even larger defects, however, the thenar and cross-finger flaps remain viable options despite these known sequelae because more donor tissue can be recruited (**Figs. 4** and **5**). These various techniques are all well described in the literature.[5–12]

Table 1
Flap options for fingertip defects

Flap	Indications	Contraindications
Smaller Defects		
VY-advancement (Atasoy and colleagues)[5]	Dorsal-oblique or transverse amputations	Amputation at or proximal to the lunula
Lateral VY-advancement (Kutler)[6]	Volar-oblique or transverse amputations	Amputation at or proximal to the lunula
Lateral pulp[7]	Lateral-oblique	Amputation of more than half the distal phalanx
Larger Defects		
Homodigital neurovascular island flaps[8,9]	Distal defects ± exposed tendons	Crush or significant injury to surrounding soft tissue
Cross-finger flap[10] and reversed cross-finger flap[11]	For volar and dorsal fingertip defects, respectively	Injury to the donor finger; vasospastic conditions (eg, Raynaud and Berger diseases)
Thenar flap[12]	Index and long fingertip injury; less commonly used for ring and little fingertip injuries	Conditions that predispose to joint stiffness (eg, rheumatoid arthritis, Dupuytren contracture, connective tissue disorders)

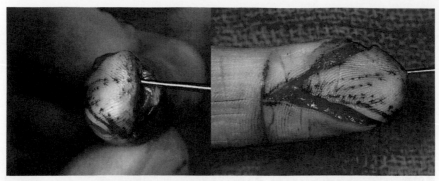

Fig. 1. Intraoperative demonstration of the degree of overcorrection necessary using the advancement flap to prevent secondary nail deformities.

When thumb defects necessitating flap coverage occur, there are several considerations involved unlike those required for similar injuries to the fingers. In addition to the need for adequate and sensate soft tissue cover of exposed bone and tendons, the critical thumb length should be preserved to maintain prehensile function without causing stiffness of the interphalangeal joint. The Moberg flap has been an excellent first choice for reconstruction of volar oblique thumb tip defects (**Fig. 6**).[13] When the wound is more extensive, the Littler flap and first dorsal metacarpal artery (FDMA) flaps are alternatives (**Figs. 7** and **8**,

Table 2)[14,15] but have less than impressive sensory restoration, which ultimately limits their utility (**Fig. 9**).[16] In contrast, the simpler-to-perform cross-finger flap based on the middle phalanges of the index and long fingers has been described as providing normal or near-normal sensibility in most patients, but its use in primary reconstruction is cautioned against due to the risk of flap ischemia from awkward positioning.[17] Dorsal thumb defects can be addressed by the reverse cross-finger flap, FDMA flap, and the Brunelli flap[18] based on the dorsoulnar artery of the thumb (**Fig. 10**).

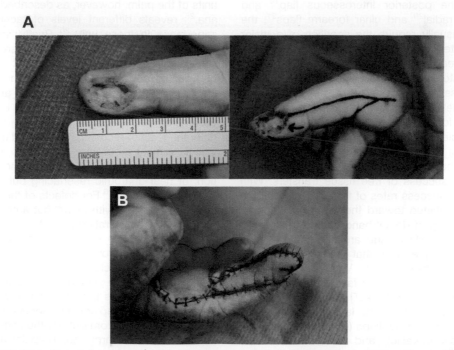

Fig. 2. (*A*) Excision of tumor from lateral nail fold and preoperative marking of a laterally based homodigital neurovascular island flap. (*B*) Final inset, providing like-for-like tissue coverage and immediate 2-point discrimination.

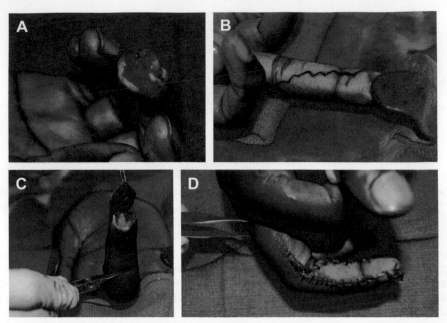

Fig. 3. (*A*) Distal fingertip injury and (*B*) design for laterally based neurovascular islanded advancement flap. (*C*) Flap harvest showing degree of potential distal advancement and (*D*) final inset of flap.

Defects of the Dorsal Hand Surface

Defects of this area include those of the dorsal hand itself, including the webspace, the wrist, and distal forearm. Local and regional flap options include the posterior interosseous flap[19] and reversed radial[20] and ulnar forearm flaps[21]; the latter 2 usually require the sacrifice of a major source artery to the hand, which may affect subsequent reconstructions and also potentially lead to cold intolerance.[22] Moreover, these flaps usually necessitate skin grafting of the donor site at an aesthetically noticeable location over the exposed forearm. Other distant options include the pedicled groin flap,[23] which has withstood the test of time, but popularity for its usage has been dwindling with the ever-expanding indications and success of free tissue transfers. With increasing success rates of free flap surgery, the focus has shifted toward the aesthetic outcome of resurfacing of dorsal hand defects because it is a cosmetically unique area characterized by thin and supple skin that is both constantly exposed and highly visible. Various options have been described, including fasciocutaneous flaps (eg, anterolateral thigh [ALT] and radial forearm), partial muscle flaps (eg, latissimus dorsi and medial rectus), fascial flaps (eg, lateral arm, ALT, and dorsal thoracic), and even venous flaps (**Fig. 11**),[24] depending on the exact soft tissue requirement for reconstruction.

Defects of the Volar Hand Surface

In general, flap coverage of palmar hand defects is addressed using the same principles as described previously. An analysis of the functional cutaneous units of the palm, however, as described by Tubiana,[25] reveals different levels of tactile gnosis importance in these units.[26] Briefly, the thenar and hypothenar eminences are considered as individual units whereas the central unit bound inbetween is considered together with the distal unit (defined by the transverse crease at the level of the interdigital folds) as one. These 3 units guide the choice of flap coverage because they have different goals of reconstruction based on an individual patient's profile—protective sensation without durability, high durability without sensation, or near-anatomic resurfacing but with poor or minor sensation.[26] For defects of the thenar or hypothenar region with or without a concomitant central deficit, restoration of protective sensation is the primary goal. This can be achieved using thin, innervated microvascular skin flaps, and local pedicled options include the radial forearm, the Becker flap, and the posterior interosseous artery flap if the forearm is spared of injury with donor nerves intact; free flap options harvested in fasciocutaneous fashion from outside the zone of injury include the lateral arm flap, scapular and parascapular flaps, thoracodorsal artery perforator flap, and ALT flap and should be coapted with an

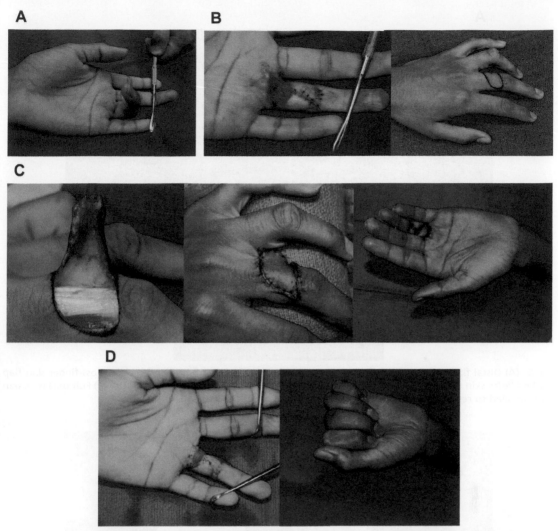

Fig. 4. (*A*) Proximal secondary volar scar contracture and (*B*) design of an oblique pattern cross-finger flap from middle finger is planned following scar release. (*C*) Cross-finger flap raised from middle finger, preserving underlying paratenon (*left*); a full-thickness skin graft is secured to the dorsal donor site (*center*) prior to inset of flap over the proximal volar defect of ring finger (*right*). (*D*) Demonstration of range of movement before division of cross-finger flap and final result after division of flap at 3 weeks.

intact sensory nerve, such as the palmar cutaneous branch of the median nerve. Combined defects of the thenar or hypothenar eminence and the central unit necessitate further consideration of patient-related factors, such as the aesthetic outcome (especially in female patients) of potential donor and recipient sites, occupation, and hand dominance to strike a balance between stable flap coverage and sensory restoration. In this instance, sensate and anatomic reconstruction is the goal and can be achieved with vascularized muscle flaps (eg, gracilis) grafted with intermediate-thickness nonglabrous skin from the plantar instep region[26]; by comparison, glabrous skin grafts may

be limited in quantity for sufficient use. Finally, for isolated defects of the combined central-distal units, mechanical stability takes precedence and is usually reconstructed with thin fascial flaps from the temporoparietal fascia, radial forearm fascia, and serratus anterior fascia.

COMPLICATIONS AND MANAGEMENT
Defects of Thumb and Fingertip Reconstruction

Bone shortening can simplify flap coverage of fingertip defects but there are several associated limitations (**Table 3**). Débridement of the distal

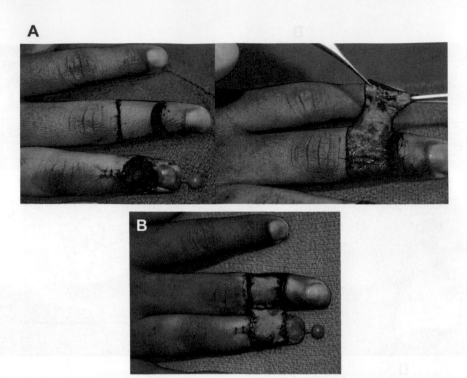

Fig. 5. (*A*) Distal fingertip wound involving the eponychial fold of ring finger and reverse cross-finger skin flap marked (*left*); skin flap raised with preservation of the nail fold on the donor finger (*right*). (*B*) Full-thickness skin graft applied to resurface adipofascial flap.

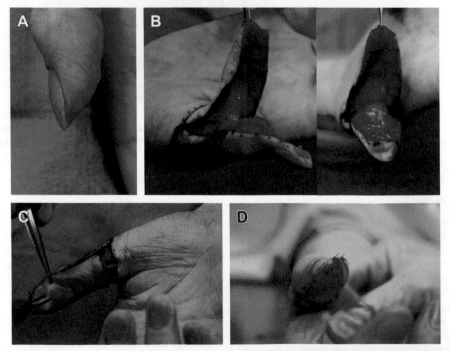

Fig. 6. (*A*) Preclinical photograph of residual thumb pulp deformity. (*B*) Moberg flap raised above the tendon sheath and (*C*) modification of traditional Moberg flap and demonstration of degree of advancement obtained from complete islanding of the flap. (*D*) Distal portion of flap is cupped and central portion of tip is allowed to granulate on final inset; proximal donor site defect may require 1 or 2 triangular flaps to achieve primary tension free closure.

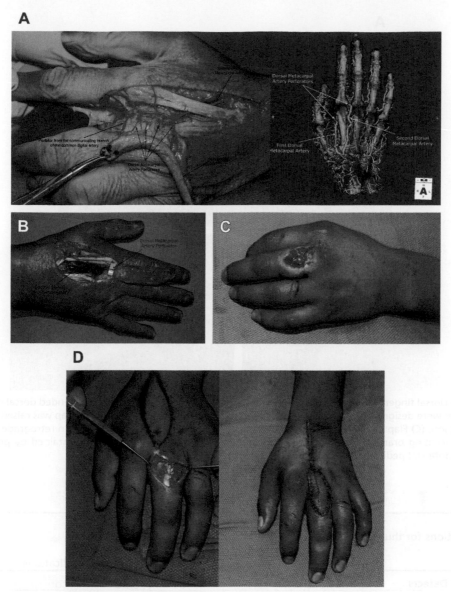

Fig. 7. (*A*) Anatomic dissection of FDMA and perforators and 3-D CT angiography of the hand and metacarpal artery perforators. (*B*) Dorsal metacarpal artery perforator dissection based on second dorsal metacarpal artery. (*C*) Traumatic injury to dorsum of middle finger involving the extensor mechanism. (*D*) Flap design planned based on dorsal metacarpal artery perforator following extensor tendon repair (*left*) and final inset of the flap (*right*), which can extend to the proximal interphalangeal joint (PIPJ).

phalanx leads to shortening and inadequate support of the overlying nail bed, which may then culminate in a hook-nail deformity as the wound heals and contracts. This may be avoided by an additional correction of 2 mm of the nail bed proximal to the terminal portion of the shortened bone (see **Fig. 1**).[27] Should débridement extend proximal to the insertion of the flexor and extensor tendons, both the aesthetic outcome due to decreased length and distal interphalangeal joint function may be affected adversely. Preservation of distal bone remnants has also been reported as a source of chronic pain and it has been suggested that for such segments less than 4 mm, they should be excised primarily at the time of injury to avoid the need for further revision procedures, such as disarticulation or amputation.[28] Other complications and their management, including venous congestion and arterial thrombosis leading to flap necrosis or loss, are well described

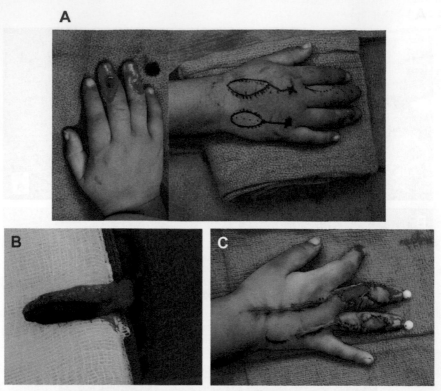

Fig. 8. (*A*) Dorsal fingertip defects at the level of the distal interphalangeal joint. (*B*) Extended dorsal metacarpal artery flaps were designed, the perforator was identified distally and divided, and the flap was raised in a retrograde fashion. (*C*) Flap inset in distal defect at distal interphalangeal joint and reliant on retrograde flow from dorsal perforating branches from the digital arteries supplying, and perfusion is maintained by preserving a broad adipofascial pedicle.

Table 2
Flap options for thumb defects

Flap	Indications	Contraindications
Smaller Defects		
Moberg[13]	Volar-oblique amputations of the thumb through distal phalanx	Usage limited to the thumb
Larger Defects		
Heterodigital neurovascular island flap (Littler)[14]	Larger defects of the volar thumb not amenable to Moberg flap	Usage limited due to poor sensory reorganization
FDMA flap[15]	Larger defects of the volar thumb not amenable to Moberg flap or dorsal defects	Usage limited due to poor sensory reorganization
Cross-finger flap[17] and reversed cross-finger flap[11]	Larger defects of the volar thumb not amenable to Moberg flap and dorsal defects, respectively	Mainly for volar-oblique hemipulp losses for the cross-finger flap
Brunelli flap[18]	Dorsal distal thumb defects or volar thumb defects	Poor sensory outcome, risk of mild webspace contracture

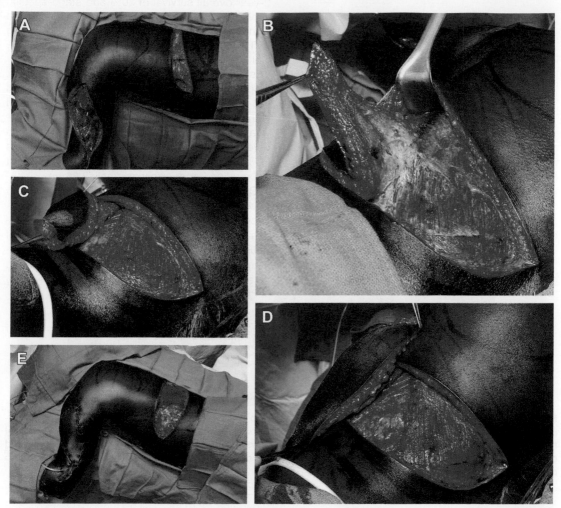

Fig. 9. Example of muscle-sparing LD for upper extremity reconstruction. (*A*) Intraoperative photograph following sarcoma excision of the lateral arm, planning of muscle-sparing latissimus dorsi muscle myocutaneous flap and incision through superior edge of skin paddle. (*B*) Skin paddle elevated medially in a subfascial plane to the border of the lateral strip of the latissimus muscle to be harvested. (*C*) Muscle sparing latissimus dorsi muscle harvested with transverse orientated skin paddle and muscle split to isolate the lateral strip of muscle only for reconstruction. (*D*) Demonstration of flap pivot and conversion to a vertical orientation without undue flap compromise, offering greater versatility prior to transfer. (*E*) Final inset for upper extremity reconstruction prior to donor site primary closure.

in the literature whereas joint stiffness and scar contractures may also occur and necessitate secondary revision procedures.

Defects of Dorsal and Volar Hand Surface Reconstruction

Complications associated with dorsal and volar hand reconstruction depend on the type of flap used. Depending on the level of harvest (axial or perforator), local pedicled flaps based on the forearm may lead to the loss of the integrity of the blood supply to the hand, so a preoperative Allen test is always indicated. This is especially important in trauma patients with compromise of the palmar

arch. Furthermore, pedicled flaps, such as the groin flap, necessitate an obligatory period of immobilization, which can lead to further joint stiffness and impair the rehabilitation process. In terms of free flap reconstruction, anastomotic thrombosis is the most frequently encountered and either requires a trial of anticoagulant therapy for example using aspirin, heparin, dextran, or prostaglandin E1, among other agents or necessitates surgical exploration and refashioning of the anastomosis or even the performance of an entirely new set of anastomosis using freshly dissected vessels. Other possible complications include those associated with the donor site, such as wound dehiscence and hematoma, which was

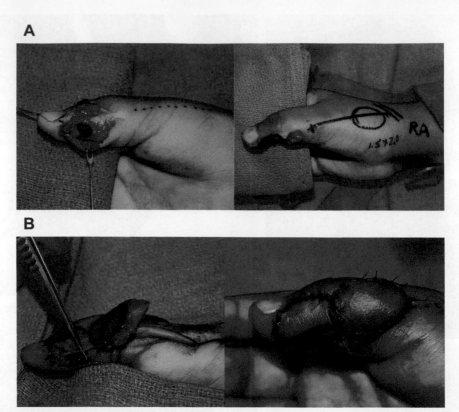

Fig. 10. (*A*) A sensitized dorsal radial artery flap of the thumb was designed after excision of a vascular malformation involving radial thumb pulp. (*B*) Flap raised with a broad pedicle, with inclusion of branch of superficial radial sensory nerve, for primary neurosynthesis, dissection carried out above the extensor paratenon and based on retrograde flow from communicating branches from the digital arteries, and inset of flap to distal thumb defect and full-thickness skin graft applied.

found in 9.5% and 2.4% of fasciocutaneous flaps in a series of 125 flaps for dorsal hand coverage.[29]

POSTOPERATIVE CARE

Free flap monitoring protocols vary between institutions but, in general, clinical bedside monitoring supersedes the various adjunctive tools that have become available, including Doppler ultrasound or laser probes, implantable perivascular devices, and percutaneous oxygen probes. Once the viability of the flap has been confirmed, hand therapy rehabilitation is initiated but with special precaution taken to avoid compression of the vascular pedicle through the use of specialized splint constructs or even external fixators to allow controlled, range-of-motion exercises similar to those after conventional tendon repairs.

OUTCOMES

Functional outcome studies after flap reconstruction of the hand are unfortunately scarce in the literature. The inherent difficulty associated with such analysis is the heterogeneity of the nature of the soft tissue defect with varying degrees of involvement of underlying skeletal, tendinous, and neurovascular injuries necessitating different treatments. Moreover, the comfort level and repertoire of flap options available invariably are highly differentiated between different surgeons depending on their levels of experience and training. A review of the available literature suggests, however, that in most cases, good outcomes can be achieved. Atasoy and colleagues[5] were able to achieve near-normal range of motion and sensory restoration in 92% of patients but the results from smaller series were less promising, with the incidence of postoperative pain and cold intolerance comparable with other methods for fingertip repair.[13,30,31] For thumb reconstruction with the Moberg flap, near-normal sensibility, defined as a 2-point discrimination of 2 mm compared with the contralateral side, and rates of postoperative pain and cold intolerance were again comparable with other procedures for the same purpose; flexion contractures of the

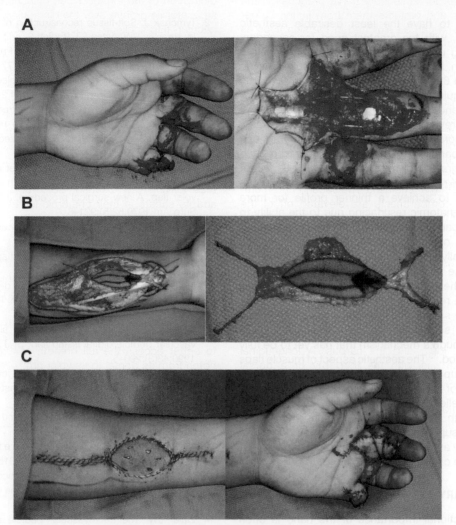

Fig. 11. (*A*) Traumatic crush injury to volar surface of right middle, ring, and little fingers, with flexor tendon injury; digital nerve segmental loss repaired with digital nerve grafts and soft tissue deficit. (*B*) Arterialized venous flap on volar forearm harvested in a suprafascial plane with 2 veins for inflow and outflow. (*C*) Final inset and full-thickness skin graft to donor site.

thumb interphalangeal joint are also rare, with less than 5° of extension loss detected, and most cases were able to sustain a full range of motion in thumbs that were normal preoperatively.[32,33] The results of sensory restoration in the Littler and

FMDA flaps are limited at best, with 2-point discrimination at 9.0 mm and 10.8 mm and cortical reorganization at 50% and 61%, respectively.[16,34] For free flap reconstruction of the dorsal and volar hand surfaces, fasciocutaneous flaps have been

Table 3
Complications and management of bone shortening in fingertip reconstruction

Complications	Management
• Hook-nail deformity • Overshortened bone segment leading to poor aesthetic outcome, distal interphalangeal joint dysfunction, chronic pain	• Excise nail bed to 2 mm proximal to débrided distal phalanx • If remnant segment <4 mm, primary excision is advocated for or else secondary procedures, such as disarticulation or excisional amputation, may be required

reported to have the least desirable aesthetic outcome, with the greatest need for secondary debulking procedures due to color and contour mismatch. In a series by Parrett and colleagues,[29] 88% and 62% of the ALT and radial forearm free flaps required further thinning procedures after dorsal hand coverage and ALT flaps needed at least 2 revisions in spite of primary thinning. Furthermore, the poor cosmetic outcome can also be partially attributed to the increased need for skin grafting of the donor site, with figures of up to 40% reported.[29] In contrast, free muscle flaps are able to achieve a thinner profile for more optimal anatomic resurfacing due to the ability to harvest partial muscle flaps for better sizing and because of postoperative denervation atrophy. Additionally, partial muscle harvest allows the avoidance of donor-site associated morbidity, such as hernias in abdomen-based flaps, and for definitive reconstruction in a 1-stage procedure. Although sensory coaptation is impossible, deep pressure sensibility may be restored in muscle flaps through a mechanism that has yet to be fully understood.[35] The aesthetic aspect of muscle flaps is also superior because its vascularity promotes the take of full-thickness skin grafts with the resultant excellent color match. By extension, fascial flaps with skin grafting and venous flaps can achieve superior outcomes in terms of donor-site morbidity and should be used with the right indications and circumstances.[36,37]

SUMMARY

The functional importance of the hand is often underestimated but there has been an increasing recognition for this rapidly expanding and particularly challenging area of reconstructive surgery. A multitude of flaps have been described and reported for various indications to meet the differing needs of patients and the responsibility lies with operating surgeons to deliberate on currently available evidence and personal experience to come up with a sound reconstructive plan that will restore, as much as possible, both form and function to a level acceptable to the patients and in the most cost-effective manner with regard to operative times, length of hospitalization, number of secondary or staged procedures, and ultimately time to functional recovery.

REFERENCES

1. Friedrich JB, Katolik LI, Vedder NB. Soft tissue reconstruction of the hand. J Hand Surg Am 2009; 34(6):1148–55.

2. Tymchak J. Soft-tissue reconstruction of the hand. In: Beasley RW, Aston SJ, Bartlett S, editors. Grabb and Smith's plastic surgery. 6th edition. Philadelphia: Lippincott Williams & Wilkins; 2007. p. 771–80.

3. Beasley RW. Principles of soft tissue replacement for the hand. J Hand Surg Am 1983;8(5 Pt 2):781–4.

4. Tonkin MA, Ahmad TS. The reconstruction of a dorsal digital defect using a reverse homodigital island flap incorporating vascularized tendon. J Hand Surg Br 1997;22(6):750–1.

5. Atasoy E, Ioakimidis E, Kasdan ML, et al. Reconstruction of the amputated finger tip with a triangular volar flap. A new surgical procedure. J Bone Joint Surg Am 1970;52(5):921–6.

6. Kutler W. A new method for finger tip amputation. J Am Med Assoc 1947;133(1):29.

7. Elliot D, Jigjinni VS. The lateral pulp flap. J Hand Surg Br 1993;18(4):423–6.

8. Lai CS, Lin SD, Yang CC. The reverse digital artery flap for fingertip reconstruction. Ann Plast Surg 1989;22(6):495–500.

9. Kojima T, Tsuchida Y, Hirasé Y, et al. Reverse vascular pedicle digital island flap. Br J Plast Surg 1990;43(3):290–5.

10. Cohen BE, Cronin ED. An innervated cross-finger flap for fingertip reconstruction. Plast Reconstr Surg 1983;72(5):688–97.

11. Pakiam AI. The reversed dermis flap. Br J Plast Surg 1978;31(2):131–5.

12. Meals RA, Brody GS. Gatewood and the first thenar pedicle. Plast Reconstr Surg 1984;73:315–9.

13. Moberg E. Aspects of sensation in reconstructive surgery of the upper extremity. J Bone Joint Surg Am 1964;46:817–25.

14. Littler JW. The neurovascular pedicle method of digital transposition for reconstruction of the thumb. Plast Reconstr Surg 1953;12(5):303–19.

15. Holevich J. A new method of restoring sensibility to the thumb. J Bone Joint Surg Br 1963;45:496–502.

16. Tränkle M, Sauerbier M, Heitmann C, et al. Restoration of thumb sensibility with the innervated first dorsal metacarpal artery island flap. J Hand Surg Am 2003;28(5):758–66.

17. Woon CY, Lee JY, Teoh LC. Resurfacing hemipulp losses of the thumb: the cross finger flap revisited: indications, technical refinements, outcomes, and long-term neurosensory recovery. Ann Plast Surg 2008;61(4):385–91.

18. Brunelli F, Vigasio A, Valenti P, et al. Arterial anatomy and clinical application of the dorsoulnar flap of the thumb. J Hand Surg Am 1999;24(4):803–11.

19. Zancolli EA, Angrigiani C. Posterior interosseous island forearm flap. J Hand Surg Br 1988;13(2):130–5.

20. Lin SD, Lai CS, Chiu CC. Venous drainage in the reverse forearm flap. Plast Reconstr Surg 1984; 74(4):508–12.

21. Guimberteau JC, Goin JL, Panconi B, et al. The reverse ulnar artery forearm island flap in hand surgery: 54 cases. Plast Reconstr Surg 1988;81(6):925–32.

22. Richardson D, Fisher SE, Vaughan ED, et al. Radial forearm flap donor-site complications and morbidity: a prospective study. Plast Reconstr Surg 1997; 99(1):109–15.

23. Heath PM, Jackson IT, Cooney WP 3rd, et al. Simultaneous bilateral staged groin flaps for coverage of mutilating injuries of the hand. Ann Plast Surg 1983;11(6):462–8.

24. Woo SH, Kim KC, Lee GJ, et al. A retrospective analysis of 154 arterialized venous flaps for hand reconstruction: an 11-year experience. Plast Reconstr Surg 2007;119(6):1823–38.

25. Tubiana R. Functional anatomy. In: Tubiana R, Mackin E, Thomine JM, editors. Examination of the hand and wrist. 2nd edition. London: Martin Dunitz; 1996. p. 1–156.

26. Engelhardt TO, Rieger UM, Schwabegger AH, et al. Functional resurfacing of the palm: flap selection based on defect analysis. Microsurgery 2012; 32(2):158–66.

27. Kumar VP, Satku K. Treatment and prevention of "hook nail" deformity with anatomic correlation. J Hand Surg Am 1993;18(4):617–20.

28. Gross SC, Watson HK. Revision of painful distal tip amputations. Orthopedics 1989;12(12):1561–4.

29. Parrett BM, Bou-Merhi JS, Buntic RF, et al. Refining outcomes in dorsal hand coverage: consideration of aesthetics and donor-site morbidity. Plast Reconstr Surg 2010;126(5):1630–8.

30. Elliot D, Moiemen NS, Jigjinni VS. The neurovascular Tranquilli-Leali flap. J Hand Surg Br 1995; 20(6):815–23.

31. O'Brien B. Neurovascular island pedicle flaps for terminal amputations and digital scars. Br J Plast Surg 1968;21(3):258–61.

32. Rohrich RJ, Antrobus SD. Volar advancement flaps. In: Blair WF, editor. Techniques in hand surgery. Baltimore (MD): Williams & Wilkins; 1996. p. 39–47.

33. Macht SD, Watson HK. The Moberg volar advancement flap for digital reconstruction. J Hand Surg Am 1980;5(4):372–6.

34. Oka Y. Sensory function of the neurovascular island flap in thumb reconstruction: comparison of original and modified procedures. J Hand Surg Am 2000; 25(4):637–43.

35. Ducic I, Hung V, Dellon AL. Innervated free flaps for foot reconstruction: a review. J Reconstr Microsurg 2006;22(6):433–42.

36. Carty MJ, Taghinia A, Upton J. Fascial flap reconstruction of the hand: a single surgeon's 30-year experience. Plast Reconstr Surg 2010;125(3):953–62.

37. Brooks D. The "reliably unreliable" venous flap. J Hand Surg Am 2009;34(7):1361–2.

Index

Note: Page numbers of article titles are in **boldface** type.

hand.theclinics.com

United States Postal Service

Statement of Ownership, Management, and Circulation
(All Periodicals Publications Except Requestor Publications)

1. Publication Title	2. Publication Number	3. Filing Date
Hand Clinics	0 0 0 - 7 0 9	9/14/14

4. Issue Frequency	5. Number of Issues Published Annually	6. Annual Subscription Price
Feb, May, Aug, Nov	4	$390.00

7. Complete Mailing Address of Known Office of Publication (Not printer) (Street, city, county, state, and ZIP+4®)

Elsevier Inc.
360 Park Avenue South
New York, NY 10010-1710

Contact Person
Stephen R. Bushing
Telephone (Include area code)
215-239-3688

8. Complete Mailing Address of Headquarters or General Business Office of Publisher (Not printer)

Elsevier Inc., 360 Park Avenue South, New York, NY 10010-1710

9. Full Names and Complete Mailing Addresses of Publisher, Editor, and Managing Editor (Do not leave blank)

Publisher (Name and complete mailing address)

Linda Belfus, Elsevier Inc., 1600 John F. Kennedy Blvd., Suite 1800, Philadelphia, PA 19103-2899

Editor (Name and complete mailing address)

Jennifer Flynn-Briggs, Elsevier Inc., 1600 John F. Kennedy Blvd., Suite 1800, Philadelphia, PA 19103-2899

Managing Editor (Name and complete mailing address)

Adrianne Brigido, Elsevier Inc., 1600 John F. Kennedy Blvd., Suite 1800, Philadelphia, PA 19103-2899

10. Owner (Do not leave blank. If the publication is owned by a corporation, give the name and address of the corporation immediately followed by the names and addresses of all stockholders owning or holding 1 percent or more of the total amount of stock. If not owned by a corporation, give the names and addresses of the individual owners. If owned by a partnership or other unincorporated firm, give its name and address as well as those of each individual owner. If the publication is published by a nonprofit organization, give its name and address.)

Full Name	Complete Mailing Address
Wholly owned subsidiary of	1600 John F. Kennedy Blvd., Ste. 1800
Reed/Elsevier, US holdings	Philadelphia, PA 19103-2899

11. Known Bondholders, Mortgagees, and Other Security Holders Owning or Holding 1 Percent or More of Total Amount of Bonds, Mortgages, or Other Securities. If none, check box ☐ None

Full Name	Complete Mailing Address
N/A	

12. Tax Status (For completion by nonprofit organizations authorized to mail at nonprofit rates) (Check one)
The purpose, function, and nonprofit status of this organization and the exempt status for federal income tax purposes:
☐ Has Not Changed During Preceding 12 Months
☐ Has Changed During Preceding 12 Months (Publisher must submit explanation of change with this statement)

PS Form 3526, August 2012 (Page 1 of 3 (Instructions Page 3)) PSN 7530-01-000-9931 PRIVACY NOTICE: See our Privacy policy in www.usps.com

---

13. Publication Title	14. Issue Date for Circulation Data Below
Hand Clinics	August 2014

15. Extent and Nature of Circulation			Average No. Copies Each Issue During Preceding 12 Months	No. Copies of Single Issue Published Nearest to Filing Date
a. Total Number of Copies (Net press run)			1,079	897
b. Paid Circulation (By Mail and Outside the Mail)	(1)	Mailed Outside-County Paid Subscriptions Stated on PS Form 3541. (Include paid distribution above nominal rate, advertiser's proof copies, and exchange copies)	710	546
	(2)	Mailed In-County Paid Subscriptions Stated on PS Form 3541 (Include paid distribution above nominal rate, advertiser's proof copies, and exchange copies)		
	(3)	Paid Distribution Outside the Mails Including Sales Through Dealers and Carriers, Street Vendors, Counter Sales, and Other Paid Distribution Outside USPS®	181	189
	(4)	Paid Distribution by Other Classes Mailed Through the USPS (e.g. First-Class Mail®)		
c. Total Paid Distribution (Sum of 15b (1), (2), (3), and (4))			891	735
d. Free or Nominal Rate Distribution (By Mail and Outside the Mail)	(1)	Free or Nominal Rate Outside-County Copies Included on PS Form 3541	34	47
	(2)	Free or Nominal Rate In-County Copies Included on PS Form 3541		
	(3)	Free or Nominal Rate Copies Mailed at Other Classes Through the USPS (e.g. First-Class Mail)		
	(4)	Free or Nominal Rate Distribution Outside the Mail (Carriers or other means)		
e. Total Free or Nominal Rate Distribution (Sum of 15d (1), (2), (3) and (4))			34	47
f. Total Distribution (Sum of 15c and 15e)			925	782
g. Copies not Distributed (See instructions to publishers #4 (page #3))			154	115
h. Total (Sum of 15f and g)			1,079	897
i. Percent Paid (15c divided by 15f times 100)			96.32%	93.99%

16. Total circulation includes electronic copies. Report circulation on PS Form 3526-X worksheets.

17. Publication of Statement of Ownership
If the publication is a general publication, publication of this statement is required. Will be printed in the November 2014 issue of this publication.

18. Signature and Title of Editor, Publisher, Business Manager, or Owner

Stephen R. Bushing – Inventory Distribution Coordinator

Date
September 14, 2014

I certify that all information furnished on this form is true and complete. I understand that anyone who furnishes false or misleading information on this form or who omits material or information requested on the form may be subject to criminal sanctions (including fines and imprisonment) and/or civil sanctions (including civil penalties).

PS Form 3526, August 2012 (Page 2 of 3)

Moving?

Make sure your subscription moves with you!

To notify us of your new address, find your **Clinics Account Number** (located on your mailing label above your name), and contact customer service at:

Email: journalscustomerservice-usa@elsevier.com

800-654-2452 (subscribers in the U.S. & Canada)
314-447-8871 (subscribers outside of the U.S. & Canada)

Fax number: 314-447-8029

Elsevier Health Sciences Division
Subscription Customer Service
3251 Riverport Lane
Maryland Heights, MO 63043

*To ensure uninterrupted delivery of your subscription, please notify us at least 4 weeks in advance of move.

Moving?

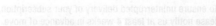

Printed and bound by CPI Group (UK) Ltd, Croydon, CR0 4YY

03/10/2024

01040376-0007